INTERMITTENT FASTING FOR WOMEN OVER OVER 50

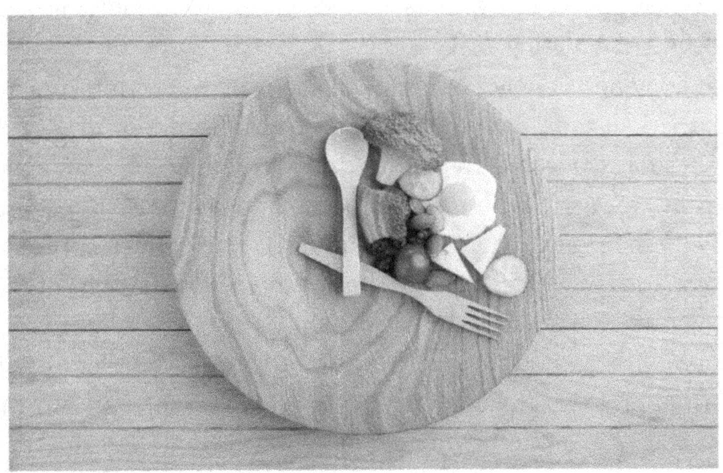

The Ultimate Guide to Lose Weight, Reset your Metabolism, Increase your Energy, Rejuvenate and Feel Better. Includes The Complete Guide for Natural Weight Loss

Mary De Blasio

I am overjoyed that you took time out of your crazy schedule to buy this book. We appreciate your efforts! The following chapters will educate you on this topic, including how intermittent fasting is not a new fad but has been around for a very long time. This book delves into the details of intermittent fasting methods, allowing you to weigh your options when it comes to fasting and losing those extra pounds. Each recipe in this book is tailored to your ketogenic low-carbohydrate diet plan. However, it is so much more than that. It also has a plethora of other health benefits.

Intermittent fasting has gained prominence in recent years, in part due to its ability to increase the rate of nutrient absorption from the foods you consume. It has also gained popularity because it does not require followers to drastically alter the types of foods they consume or the times of day they consume them. It does not even require a significant change in the amount of calories consumed in a 24-hour period. Indeed, the most popular form of intermittent fasting is simply eating two slightly larger-than-average meals during the day rather than the standard three.

This makes the intermittent fasting diet plan an ideal option for those who struggle to adhere to more restrictive diet plans, since it requires only one habit change—the amount of meals a day—rather than many. Numerous individuals discover that intermittent fasting produces tangible results. It's easy enough to sustain over time and effective enough to produce the sort of results that can sustain motivation long after the novelty wears off.

The key to intermittent fasting's effectiveness is that your body reacts differently when you're fasting than when you're eating. When you are in a fed state, the body is constantly digesting and consuming food. This process starts approximately five minutes after you finish eating and will last between three and five hours, depending on how difficult the food is for your body to digest. When you are eating, your body is constantly releasing insulin, impairing your body's ability to burn fat properly.

During the time after digestion, insulin levels start falling back to normal, which can take anywhere between eight to 12 hours. This is the transition state between the fed and fasted states. The fasting state starts when your insulin levels return to normal. This is the optimal time for your body to process fat. Unfortunately, since people seldom go eight hours, let alone twelve, without any kind of caloric intake, many people never reach a point where they can efficiently burn fat.

There is reason to be hopeful! To begin seeing real results, however, you must break the three-meal-a-day routine.

Adhere to the intermittent fasting guidelines outlined in this insightful book. Additionally, you will discover numerous new tips and instructions in each chapter. By the end of the book, you'll understand how to prepare healthy meals while adhering to the fasting protocol, thanks to the delicious recipes included in the later chapters. You can prepare healthy breakfast, lunch, and dinnertime meals using your Instant Pot, Crock-Pot, stovetop, or microwave, or any other food appliance. As you will quickly discover, this endeavour is not nearly as difficult as you believe!

There are numerous books on this topic available on the market, so thank you for selecting this one! Every effort has been made to ensure that it is as comprehensive as possible. Please take advantage of each subject to the fullest!

Although losing weight is a necessity, few people consider the benefits of weight loss or how diets and diet plans are not created solely for the purpose of weight loss. Consider intermittent fasting. The majority of people believe that intermittent fasting is an easy, no-effort way to lose weight and fat. However, have you considered its additional health benefits or the fact that it is not a "weight loss programme," but rather a shift in your eating schedule that results in weight loss?

I'll discuss what intermittent fasting is and how you, as a woman, can get the most value from it in this book. The majority of intermittent fasting programmes are geared toward or tailored for males. These plans often overlook the fact that women need a shorter fasting duration or the effect of intermittent fasting on the body's hormonal balance. However, in this book, women are the focus, and all of the material is geared toward assisting you in successfully adjusting to intermittent fasting!

CHAPTER 1: INTERMITTENT FASTING: WHAT YOU NEED TO KNOW

Fasting is not a modern concept. For a significant portion of human existence, humans have fasted due to food shortages or religious/spiritual purposes. Nowadays, people fast far less than in the past, which makes sense given the abundance of food available. On the other hand, intermittent fasting is a relatively recent concept. It's a novel and distinct method of meal preparation. Intermittent fasting has been shown to have a number of health and longevity benefits. It has shown that when done correctly, it can help us control our body weight, prolong our lives, and regulate our blood glucose levels, among other benefits.

We are used to eating three meals a day and possibly snacking in between. However, Intermittent Fasting is distinct. Intermittent Fasting is a deliberate decision to forego those meals. This can be done once a week, or it can mean skipping breakfast entirely and making lunch your first meal of the day. There are many ways to do this, but it truly depends on the objectives.

Intermittent Fasting is a term that refers to depriving yourself of food at specific times of the day. You can eat only during specific hours, referred to as 'Time Windows.' You will choose these time windows based on what works best for you during the day. For instance, if you want to eat between 12:00 PM and 8:00 PM, that is your time window. You'll ensure that you eat all of your calories during those hours and not at any other time.

It is also up to you how many meals you consume. You can choose to split your food into five or six meals, or you can consume either one or two meals. Regardless, the central principle is the same: eating all of your calories within a specified time period (your time window).

Thus, Intermittent Fasting is not a diet; rather, it is a method of eating calories in a particular way. It has nothing to do with the food you consume, but rather with the time you consume it. To be well, of course, you must eat healthy foods and avoid overeating in the first place, but Intermittent Fasting itself has many benefits.

Numerous studies have shown Intermittent Fasting's health benefits. According to one study conducted on rats, fasting increased the rats' lifespan by 10% to 20% as compared to rats that did not fast. Another research demonstrated that Intermittent Fasting increases longevity and susceptibility to many age-related diseases.

Additionally, it demonstrated that it greatly enhances the health of obese humans. It also indicated that the benefits are comparable to those associated with calorie restriction.

INTERMITTENT FASTING: THE SCIENCE

When you eat, your body responds differently than when you fast. When you consume food, the body can absorb it within a few hours. The meal would be burned off as food for the body, with the remainder being retained as fat. However, with Intermittent Fasting, the situation is reversed. When you fast, your body will burn previously stored body fat for fuel rather than the meals you consume. This is because your body will always take the simplest path, and if there is no food available, it will draw energy from fat stores.

One of the most common errors people make when beginning to practise Intermittent Fasting is believing they can consume as much food as they want. This, however, is incorrect! Again, the central concept of Intermittent Fasting is to consume all of your calories during specific hours (your time window). This does not mean that you can consume more (or less) food than normal. It basically means that you will consume all of your meals during specific hours and will abstain from eating anything else during those hours. Therefore, if you've been fasting for some time but aren't seeing results on the scale, this may mean one of two things:

1) You consume an excessive amount of food.

The following is a straightforward formula for weight loss: Weight loss = consuming less calories than you burn. I'm not concerned about how many hours you spend on the treadmill or how many miles you run each day. Each day, you must burn more calories than you eat. Everybody burns a certain number of calories daily, as the body needs calories to work properly. You must ensure that you eat less calories than you burn on a daily basis. Intermittent fasting, weight conditioning, cardio, and sports are just a few examples. All of these things will help you lose weight faster, but they are not the fundamentals! If you fail to adhere to the fundamentals (consuming less calories than you burn off), you are still struggling to lose weight.

2) You are obtaining results but are unaware of them.

I've had a number of clients who were disappointed by their inability to see any improvement. I will inquire of them, "How do you evaluate yourself?" The majority of them responded, "I weigh myself daily / weekly by standing on the scale." And nine times out of ten, they would already be seeing results but were unaware.

The scale is an inherently imperfect method of measurement. This is because the weight on the scale indicates not just how much fat you have stored, but also how much water, food, and muscle you have consumed. Thus, it is possible that you are seeing results but are unaware of them since you have consumed a large amount of water, developed muscle, and/or recently consumed a meal. To accurately calculate yourself, you must do so weekly at the same time. Additionally, you will need additional measuring instruments in addition to your scale. To determine your fat percentage, you'll need fat clippers and a measuring tape. And how do you gauge your own worth? Utilize the fat clippers to determine the amount of fat on your body and the measuring tape to determine the amount of fat on each part of your body (arms, legs, belly, etc.).

Having said that, the concepts outlined in this book will yield the best results when combined with a healthy diet. This includes consuming the right foods, avoiding excessive calorie consumption, and removing unhealthy foods from your diet. It is implausible to expect results from Intermittent Fasting when maintaining an unhealthy diet.

GOING FURTHER

When we feed, our bodies release insulin, which acts as a signal for the foods we eat to be converted to glycogen or fat. Fasting reduces insulin levels, signalling the body that it wants to use fat reserves for food. As a result, the body receives a significant metabolic boost in a number of ways.

Rest and rejuvenation

To begin, by abstaining from food, you allow your internal organs to cleanse themselves of wastes and toxins, increasing the efficiency of your internal engine. It's the equivalent to changing the air filter in your furnace. Suddenly, the house feels colder, and the heater doesn't have to work as hard to keep everyone inside.

According to experts, a healthy liver is critical for proper metabolism, so giving it a break for a few hours helps it to flush out contaminants that cause it to feel overworked and get back to work on the job it was designed to do. Following a fast, the colon walls are cleansed of impacted faeces, allowing for improved nutrient absorption. Additionally, the pancreas, gall bladder, and liver regenerate and thereby metabolise food more efficiently

The amount of Human Growth Hormone increases.

After 18 hours of fasting, the body produces elevated amounts of human growth hormone, providing a significant boost to muscles. Fasting stimulates the development of growth hormone, which prevents muscle loss during the fast. As a result, the metabolism increases, owing primarily to the fact that muscle is responsible for the majority of metabolism. After 36 hours of fasting, the metabolism begins to slow.

Incentive programmes for weight loss

When the body runs out of glucose to use as fuel during a short, it immediately turns to fat stores for energy. In a way, forcing the body to use the fat cell bank retrains it, making it more likely to use stored fat cells during times of normal feeding. Indeed, fasting for 24 hours increases the amount of fat released from fat reserves and the amount of fat burned for fuel by about 50%. Doubling fat burn is a simple way to lose excess weight and reveal a leaner physique.

Regulation of blood sugar and insulin

Insulin is present to assist the body in processing carbohydrates and fats and in storing excess calories as fat. Insulin resistance develops over time, requiring an increasing amount of insulin to absorb the same amount of food. Increased insulin levels result in increased fat storage, which is one of the reasons why experts believe it becomes more difficult to lose weight as we age.

Fasting on an intermittent basis interrupts the loop.

During a fast, the body burns fat slowly and steadily, ensuring that blood sugar and insulin levels remain stable, without the spikes associated with many dieters' energy highs and lows. A 2003 research on mice discovered that mice that were subjected to intermittent fasting that mimicked calorie restriction had lower blood glucose and insulin levels, leading the study's authors to conclude that intermittent fasting has beneficial effects on glucose control. The increased insulin sensitivity is critical because the benefits last long after the fast is completed, making it more difficult to gain weight in the future.

Experts also discovered that there is a plethora of advantages to be gained by building on our ancestors' experiences and using intermittent fasting. One of the most significant advantages is comparable to those of people who follow a carb-free or low-carbohydrate diet.

Going without food for an extended period of time forces the body to burn fat reserves for fuel rather than the glucose produced when the foods we consume are converted into glucose. Fasting, in essence, results in the burning of excess fat, which practically melts away. Your metabolism will not slow, you will not lose muscle, your workouts will not suffer, and you will not transform into a ravenous eater.

Food Stress Has Been Eliminated

Food will no longer be a constant source of worry during the day. I believe that eating every three hours, cycling your protein and carbohydrate intake, and monitoring your glycemic index are not enough for sustained weight loss. Food and feeding would no longer be an obsessive-compulsive act with intermittent fasting.

Other supporters concur that one of the primary advantages of intermittent fasting is relieving food-related tension. I didn't waste any time contemplating or obsessing about when or how my next meal would arrive. Worrying about such stuff had been my normal mode of operation for a long period of time after I became more interested in my training and diet, and it was a relief to no longer have to expend any mental energy on it.

Food As Fuel

Rather than thinking about what to eat and what to eat, the time spent fasting can be used to prepare meals that will provide the body with the most food. To me, life is not about eating in order to survive, but rather about living in order to eat. With intermittent fasting, I was no longer plagued by achy knees, daytime exhaustion, mental fogs, and other ailments that harmed my work and athletic results. I believe that I could be healthier at 36 than I was at 26.

Finally, You Will Feel Aware and Awake Without the peaks and valleys associated with blood sugar spikes caused by consuming the wrong foods at the wrong times, energy levels remain consistent throughout the day. Additionally, many intermittent fasting practitioners report that the diet offers a sense of consistency that they lacked when food was weighing them down.

Many people report improved mental clarity and increased energy following a brief fast. Contrary to common opinion, fasting does not result in a decline in mental performance or energy. However, the human body is an incredible and highly adaptable machine, and the notion that it will begin to shut down in the short term due to a lack of food is nonsense. After all, how could our forefathers and mothers have survived those long winters of scarce food if their bodies shut down before they could find something edible?

Muscle Tone Enhancement

Intermittent fasting does not harm the muscles because it burns stored fat for fuel, helping you to push through your workouts with ease. The critical point is to ensure that you break your fast and consume a recovery meal within 30 minutes of exercising. Protein is needed by the body to regenerate muscles and repair damage sustained during the workout. By skipping the vital meal, you put yourself in danger of injury.

Cleansed And Refreshed Fasting provides the body with a break from food digestion, enabling it to focus on cleaning itself of toxins that accelerate our ageing process.

By fasting, you are assisting Mother Nature in eliminating the toxins and wastes that have accumulated in your body. Fasting increases the rate of waste removal from dead and damaged cells, a process called autophagy. Autophagy's inability to keep up with accumulated cellular debris is widely believed to be a significant cause of chronic diseases associated with ageing."

Increased Life Expectancy

In the early 1900s, a variety of research examining the health benefits of calorie restriction discovered that reducing daily caloric intake by 30% could help us live longer while decreasing our risk of developing a variety of different health problems, including diabetes, blood clots, Alzheimer's, heart failure, and a variety of other diseases.

Since intermittent fasting can imitate the benefits of calorie restriction, it offers the same benefits without the negative health consequences associated with calorie restriction. Fasting is often analogous to shutting down and cleaning a complex and useful computer in order for it to operate more efficiently and effectively. Resting the gastrointestinal tract, enabling cells and tissues to rebuild themselves, and allowing the lymph, blood, and organs to eliminate old, deficient, or diseased cells and unnecessary chemicals all contribute to decreased degeneration and sickness. As healthy cell growth is enhanced, our fertility, immune function, and disease tolerance, as well as our capacity for longer life, are increased.

While many people believe that depriving oneself of food for an extended period of time is unhealthy, scientists have shown that Intermittent Fasting has numerous benefits. I will demonstrate the benefits of Intermittent Fasting in this chapter.

1. It eliminates food/sugar cravings

Oftentimes, when we feel "hungry," we are really craving sugars and carbohydrates. When you hard, your body switches from carbohydrate to fat-burning mode. Your body will eventually discover that carbohydrates are not needed for energy and that it can generate energy from the fat already stored in your body. Apart from eliminating sugar cravings, you can also eliminate food cravings. Since your body "realises" that it does not need food for energy, it will not crave it as much. Thus, by eliminating all hunger stimuli, you will be able to get through the day.

This is why the theory of "eating five or six times a day" is false. When you consume food five to six times a day and include carbohydrates, you will never cause your body to burn fat. This is because the body can first use the carbohydrates in your body for energy before it uses the fat in your body.

2. It increases insulin sensitivity

Insulin is a hormone produced by the body that controls cell function. The pancreas produces insulin, which is secreted when we feed. It then interacts with signalling cells, allowing our bodies to store sugars as energy. The less insulin we need to store these sugars, the more insulin sensitive we become, and the more effectively insulin can perform its function over time.

When we eat five to six times a day, our insulin levels remain abnormally elevated for an extended period of time. This insulin would be ineffective, ultimately increasing our resistance to it. When the body becomes immune to insulin, type 2 diabetes or prediabetes may develop. Diabetes is a condition in which we are unable to store all of the sugars we eat because the insulin produced by our pancreas is ineffective.

When this occurs, the sugars are not converted to energy and remain in our blood stream, resulting in elevated blood sugar levels and vessel hardening. This can potentially result in kidney failure, heart attacks, erectile dysfunction, vision loss, strokes, and nerve damage, among other serious health complications. When you fast for an extended period of time, though, you force your body to burn stored fat for energy rather than the food you are digesting. This will allow your body to produce less insulin and thus become more insulin responsive, thus avoiding all of these complications.

3. It is extremely simple

Intermittent fasting is a relatively simple concept. Planning the amount, consistency, and timing of your meals does not take much effort. Many regular gym goers go to great lengths to prepare their meals in order to keep track of their calories. Although this approach is adequate in and of itself, it can be very energy- and time-consuming. Owing to the fact that we no longer have much time in this day and age due to our fast-paced, stressful lifestyles, it is preferable to save time by eliminating repetitive tasks such as meal preparation.

When you fast, you just have to think about one or two meals a day, and you still know when you're going to eat. This enables you to devote more time to more critical tasks. When you accept that meal preparation is no longer necessary, you will find that you can achieve the same results with less effort. This is often referred to as the 80/20 rule. 80% of our results are the product of 20% of our efforts. It is up to us to determine which 20% is important. Quite sometimes, meal preparation is not included in the 20%.

Additionally, since you will be consuming one or two big meals a day, you will not need to regularly monitor your calorie intake. Additionally, it is much more difficult to eat more than the daily calorie requirement in one or two meals.

This does not happen if you are a certified bodybuilder. You cannot hope to participate and win competitions if you are not as lean as possible. Therefore, for those who are competing, I strongly advise you to watch all of your calories and stick to what works!

4. It is adaptable.

Maintaining a strict meal schedule can be extremely difficult. The majority of us have critical and time-consuming occupations that prevent us from eating when we need to. Other than that, we receive breaks when we least need them. Or we are always on the move, which prevents us from eating when we need to. However, fasting allows for a great deal of versatility. Due to the limited time available, you can choose when to eat. This allows you to eat when it is most convenient for you.

When I travel or work, it becomes extremely difficult for me to prepare my meals and adhere to my meal schedule. Fasting enables me to go long periods of time without food and only eat when the time is right for me.

5. Health advantages

Numerous studies have shown the numerous health benefits of intermittent fasting. Overweight individuals and those suffering from diseases such as diabetes can benefit the most from intermittent fasting.

Individuals who are overweight or have type 2 diabetes who fast occasionally can lose more weight and boost their heart health. They will see results even though they do not reduce their calorie consumption (but rather remain in maintenance mode). However, if you want to optimise your performance, you can maintain a slight calorie deficit and consume nutritious foods.

Additionally, it has the following health benefits: It reduces inflammation

It lowers blood pressure

It improves pancreatic function

It protects against cardiovascular disease

It lowers total cholesterol and LDL levels

It improves insulin sensitivity

Nota bene: *If you are diabetic, consult your physician before beginning Intermittent Fasting! Although intermittent fasting is beneficial for diabetics in and of itself, it can be harmful if you deprive yourself of nutrients at certain times of the day. Again, if you are diabetic, intermittent fasting is beneficial, but consult your doctor first!*

6. Rapid weight loss

As previously mentioned, carbohydrates provide capacity. This will keep the body from burning the fat it has accumulated. However, when you hard, you force your body to burn stored fat for energy. This will result in immediate and rapid weight loss, which means you will not only look better, but will also be healthier.

Additionally, by fasting for one or two days a week, you are naturally consuming less calories (1000-4500 calories a week). This will result in significant and rapid weight loss, with an average of 0.5-1 pound per week! You'll be able to maintain muscle mass while losing weight, resulting in incredible body transformations.

7. **improves brain health**

Intermittent fasting also has many cognitive benefits. It enhances memory capacity and speeds up learning. Additionally, it increases the BDNF (Brain Derived Neurotrophic Factor), which helps develop brain tissues. This will improve your intelligence and assist you in developing stronger muscles.

√ **Prevents depression**
Researchers have established a correlation between low BDNF levels and depression.

√ **Beneficial in the Fight Against Alzheimer's Disease**
Two mice with Alzheimer's disease were used in the research. One mouse was on an Intermittent Fasting diet, while the other was on a normal diet (both were consuming the same amount of calories). They were placed in a Morris water maze, and the mouse observing Intermittent Fasting navigated much more quickly than the other.

√ **Increases the development of ketones**
sporadic Fasting promotes the synthesis of ketones in an active manner. Ketones are acids produced by the body to assist it in burning fat for energy rather than carbohydrates.

√ **Effective Against Traumatic Brain Injury**
Fasting alleviates mitochondrial dysfunction, oxidative stress, and cognitive impairment associated with brain trauma.

√ **Prevents the onset of Huntington's disease**

While this disease depletes BDNF levels, research has shown that fasting rats with Huntington's disease maintain stable BDNF levels.

The term autophagy is derived from the Greek words auto, which means "self," and phagein, which means "to consume." The two words together literally mean "to eat oneself." I understand how gruesome this idea sounds, but autophagy is essential for the body's optimal health. Autophagy is the process of a cell's damaged and worn-out sections being broken down and recycled. Autophagy also means that cells can survive starvation. The recycled parts are then used to reconstruct new structures inside the cell. Even though we live in an old home, we are remodeling the kitchen to make it clean, sleek, and modern.

The mammalian target of rapamycin, or mTOR for short, is responsible for autophagy. The mTOR gene is found in every cell in the body. We consider mTOR to be an insulin, amino acid, oxygen, and energy sensor. As a result, the mTOR senses that the body is consuming food as we consume carbohydrates or proteins. Since the body breaks down carbohydrates into glucose, which activates insulin secretion, the presence of mTOR signals the cells that the body has a supply of nutrients on the way. In the meantime, the digestive system breaks down proteins into amino acids, which activates the mTOR sensor. Since the body uses nutrients to create structures, the presence of mTOR inhibits autophagy.

Insulin levels drop while glucagon levels increase when a person fasts. Insulin and glucagon battle each other. Glucagon tells the muscles to release glycogen, or sugar stored in the muscles. Since there are no nutrients coming in, mTOR goes dormant and autophagy kicks in. By depleting amino acids, glucagon can also aid in the activation of autophagy. As a result, the body switches to recycle mode.

The human body is extremely complex, and autophagy can be triggered by a variety of factors. When nutrients become scarce, for example, the protein AMPK (adenosine monophosphate-activated protein kinase) rises and activates autophagy. AMPK also disables mTOR. How long does a person have to fast before autophagy kicks in? The replies range from 8 hours to three days, depending on who we ask. However, we know that liver glycogen and insulin levels drop after 12 hours of fasting, while glucagon levels peak after 13 hours. Within this time, our digestive systems would have processed and assimilated all of the protein, so mTOR would turn off while AMP would turn on, triggering autophagy. Naturally, how one's hormones respond during a fast varies from person to person.

Obese people and diabetics can also have lower levels of autophagy. Most possibly, they have high and persistent insulin levels, which prevent their bodies from turning off mTOR and, as a result, turning on autophagy.

We also have no means of measuring autophagy since it takes place inside the cells. Some fasters keep track of their insulin and glucagon levels, as well as their insulin-to-glucagon ratio. Ketone strips are used by other fasters to check the amount of ketones in their blood or urine. If the body burns ketones for food, autophagy should have been enabled. Furthermore, autophagy responds to stress on a cell, and other pathways, such as dehydration (as in a dry fast), severe heat or cold, or hypoxia (i.e., oxygen deprivation), activate autophagy. Of course, I do not recommend that fasters go without oxygen.

The mTOR pathway is extremely responsive, and only 3 grams of the amino acid leucine will stop autophagy. Intense exercise also activates autophagy by causing mTOR to go dormant. In a mouse sample, 30 minutes of treadmill running turned on AMPK and turned off mTOR. As a result, autophagy and exercise go together like soda and popcorn at the movies. That is why, during a fast, we must be cautious about what we drink. A splash of milk in our coffee can temporarily stop autophagy.

In 1974, Christian de Duve was awarded the Nobel Prize in Physiology or Medicine for discovering the mechanism of autophagy. Lysosomes, a component of any cell, are essential for autophagy. Within a cell, a lysosome functions as a stomach and contains digestive enzymes. Autophagy then allows a lysosome to release enzymes that digest aged, broken down cell pieces, including bacteria and viruses that have been engulfed. The cell then recycles the components to create new cell structures.

THERE ARE THREE TYPES OF AUTOPHAGY.

Macro-autophagy: A cell's autophagosome is formed inside the cell. It resembles a small Pac-Man that eats garbage, invading cells, and weakened cell structures as it moves around the cell. In a damaged cell, the autophagosome engulfs an organelle (or "small organ"), damaged proteins, fats (or lipids), or bacteria, and then fuses with the lysosome. The lysosome's digestive juices break down the weakened organelle into proteins, fatty acids, and raw materials, which the body will then recycle. Furthermore, during nutrient deficiency or cell stress, cells produce autophagosomes, which are essential for a person's longevity.

Fasting for short periods of time will boost the size and number of autophagosomes in cells. Scientists discovered few and tiny autophagosomes within neuron cells or brain cells in a study of well-fed male mice. The autophagosomes multiplied and grew in size after a 24-hour fasting. When compared to a well-fed state, autophagosomes grew 3 to 4 times larger and more numerous after 48 hours of fasting.

Macroautophagy is divided into two types: mitophagy and lipophagy. Mitophagy is the recycling of a cell's mitochondria. The mitochondria, also known as the cell's energy furnace, supply heat and energy to the cell. Lipophagy, on the other hand, directs autophagy to lipids, or fat.

Micro-autophagy: Inside a cell, the lysosome attaches itself directly to the cytoplasm. The cytoplasm contains all of the cell's material except the nucleus, as well as mitochondria and lipids. Microautophagy is unaffected by nutrient scarcity. It's just part of the maintenance process.

Autophagy mediated by a chaperone: A particular protein selects and binds with a material, fusing it directly to the lysosome. Within a cell, the basic protein scavenges for proteins one by one. This selective autophagy can be triggered by a nutrient deficiency, which may be essential for a person's longevity.

We can see why exercise and fasting are so important. By recycling old parts inside a cell, autophagy slows the harmful effects of aging and age-related diseases. As a result, we take our trusty old car to the mechanic for a tune-up and some repairs, and the engine purrs like a cat.

Fasting is known to encourage and induce autophagy.

The rise of ketones, especially beta-hydroxybutyrate, is thought to signal the body's cells to activate autophagy. During a fast, we can use a variety of techniques to boost autophagy and the ketosis state.

1. During a fast, we exercise to improve autophagy. Autophagy is supported by both aerobic and resistance exercise.

2. During a fast, we should drink coffee. By raising AMPK and lowering mTOR, researchers discovered that both standard and decaffeinated coffee promote autophagy in heart, liver, and muscle cells in mice.

3. We can drink green tea, which contains the polyphenol epigallocatechin gallate, during a fast (EGCG). The EGCG activates AMPK and autophagy in the liver cells of mice.

4. Sweating in saunas and shivering in ice baths may promote autophagy, which protects the body's cells from external stress. The Russians have it right when they sit in a hot sauna and then run and jump into an icy lake in the winter.

During our feasting cycle, we can use a variety of methods to improve autophagy. By triggering AMPK, the ketogenic diet, coconut oil (or medium-chain triglycerides), and supplements like berberine and resveratrol facilitate autophagy.

Intermittent fasting comes in a variety of forms. They all follow the same fundamental rules, but their implementation differs. In this chapter, I'll go through the five most popular Intermittent Fasting Models currently in use. Make sure you read the entire chapter to determine which model is best for your health goals.

1. LEANGAINS

This Intermittent Fasting variation, created by Martin Berkhan, is ideally suited for people who regularly go to the gym and want to lose weight and add muscle.

The fundamentals

You have an 8-hour time span and will fast for the next 16 hours (14 hours for women). During the fasting time, you will not eat any calories. Diet soda, calorie-free sweeteners, black coffee, tea, and sugar-free gum, on the other hand, are permitted.

Time frames

It is up to you to decide when your time window begins and ends, but it is recommended that you plan ahead and stick to your schedule. It's important to keep it sustainable, so set the time window on days and times that are convenient for you. If you go to the gym every morning, for example, it is not a good idea to eat a big meal right before you go. If you work a 9-5 job, I wouldn't suggest eating all of your calories when you're there because it will make it difficult for you to stay focused on your work. Often, we are creatures of habit, so take advantage of that. Decide ahead of time when your time window will begin each day, and stick to it! If you are inconsistent, sticking to the program would be more difficult because you are repeatedly breaking the habit and not allowing yourself the opportunity to form the habit in the first place.

Food categories

The foods you consume are determined by your goals, body weight, age, and gender. And on non-workout days, you can consume plenty of protein. However, don't eat too much because this can cause protein toxicity. While trying to lose body fat, it's crucial to consume more carbohydrates than fats on training days, but lower your total carbohydrate intake.

You can consume whole, unprocessed foods the majority of the time, regardless of your objectives. You can have cheat days now and then, but only in moderation.

It is cost effective.

When you miss those meals, such as breakfast and lunch, you will be able to save money. Many people underestimate how much money they spend per day on breakfast and lunch.

Calorie counting isn't essential

It would be incredibly difficult to consume so many calories if you want to eat in a limited time window or eat all of your calories in one or two meals (if you are not eating junk food). As a result, you can avoid the hassle of constantly monitoring your calorie intake.

Helps to burn fat

When you adopt the Leangains diet, you can naturally consume less carbohydrates than you would otherwise. This would result in a significant amount of body fat being burned. Your body can adjust to the fact that you aren't consuming a lot of carbohydrates and will burn any stored fat for energy.

The drawbacks of leangains

Leangains allows for a lot of flexibility in terms of what you eat, but it is also specific on the types of foods you should eat. The majority of the time, this would not be an issue for active gym addicts, since the most dedicated are still disciplined in their diet.

2.   THE WARRIOR DIET

Ori Hofmekler initiated the project. This is a very strict diet that is ideally suited to people who are self-disciplined. This diet encourages people to consume only one big, high-quality meal a day, with a few snacks scattered throughout the day.

The fundamentals

You'll fast for 20 hours and then eat one big meal rich in nutrients. You can't eat all you want during your time window because you need to avoid additives and combine the right foods. While fasting, you can eat small snacks such as raw fruits and vegetables, as well as drink fresh juice and eat a few servings of protein.

A few servings of protein per day will help you maximize your nervous system's "fight or flight" response. This increases alertness while also promoting fat-burning and providing energy boosts.

When we feed at night, the parasympathetic nervous system is at its best. That's why the best time to visit is at night. This will assist our bodies in remaining calm and balanced when digesting food. Another advantage of eating late at night is that it aids fat burning during the day.

During the four-hour time frame, there is often a clear order in which to feed. Vegetables should come first, followed by protein, and finally fat. You should consume some carbohydrates if you are still hungry after that meal.

THE WARRIOR DIET'S ADVANTAGES

Snacking During Fasting Periods

One of the key advantages of this diet is that you can feed during your fasting window on occasion. Fruits, vegetables, and fruit juice are all appropriate.

Excellent Health

Another advantage of this diet is that it ensures that you get all of the nutrients you need on a regular basis.

The warrior diet's drawbacks

Since it is so strict on when and when to eat, this diet can be difficult to stick to. Many citizens cannot afford to eat late at night, and some find it difficult to eat healthily on a regular basis.

Brad Pilon developed a classic Intermittent Fasting model. This is ideal for people who already eat a healthy diet but want to lose weight quickly.

The Eat Stop Eat Principles entails fasting for 24 hours once or twice a week. While fasting, you may drink calorie-free beverages. It's as though you're fasting for 24 hours and then returning to your normal diet. The trick is to ignore the fact that you fasted and go about your business as usual. Pretend you didn't easy. It is also entirely up to you if you end your fasting period with a large meal or a snack.

EAT STOP EAT'S ADVANTAGES

Calorie Deficiency Without Using Willpower

Since you're just restricting your eating for one or two days, you won't need much (or any) willpower. It will be much easier to stick to the 24-hour fast if you know you can eat anything you want after you've completed it.

Eat as much as you can

You can also eat whatever you want, whenever you want, which will help you avoid binges. The only catch is that moderation is important. Poor foods can only be consumed in moderation. It's good to have one or two hands of chips, but eating a bag of chips every day is not.

Eat stop eat's drawbacks

Even when you have complete freedom to consume whatever you want, the Eat Stop Eat diet can be difficult to stick to. Some people struggle to consume unhealthy foods in moderation or indulge on the days they are allowed to eat. If you're having trouble with self-control, I wouldn't suggest this form.

3.   THE ALTERNATE DAY DIET

James Johnson pioneered the Alternate Day Diet. Dr. Johnson had an epiphany, realizing that most people are unable to maintain a constant calorie restriction. He also noticed that his eating style had many health benefits, so he wanted to share his version of Intermittent Fasting with the rest of the world. This plan is ideal for dieters who are already disciplined and have a clear weight loss target in mind.

The fundamentals

The Alternate Day Diet works on the basic idea of eating normally one day and very little the next. On average days, you will consume your daily calorie requirement, and on low-calorie days, you will consume 20% of your daily calorie requirement. So, if your daily calorie requirement is 2000, you'll consume 2000 calories on day 1, 500 on day 2, 2000 on day 3, 500 on day 4, and so on.

Everyone's body needs a different amount of calories on a daily basis. This is determined by your age, gender, height, weight, and amount of exercise you get on a regular basis. There are a plethora of reliable resources available on the internet to assist you in determining your daily calorie requirements.

On low-calorie days, you are required to drink meal replacement shakes to make things easier. However, you can just use these shakes for the first two weeks of the diet to get the most out of it. Following that, you should eat real food. Dr. Johnson also suggests that you exercise on your regular calorie days.

THE ALTERNATIVE DAY DIET ADVANTAGES

Lose Weight Quickly

You will see results quickly because you are cutting a large number of calories per day. Many people claim to be losing 1-2 pounds each week.

Eat Your Favorite Foods

There are no dietary restrictions, but it is recommended that you consume unprocessed and whole foods. On average calorie days, however, you can only consume as many calories as you need to maintain your weight.

Doesn't necessitate a lot of willpower

You won't need much willpower because you'll only be cutting calories for 2-3 days a week. It will be difficult at first, but it is preferable to begin the diet slowly. On low-calorie days, start by reducing a small amount of calories and gradually increase it.

Eat stop eat's drawbacks

This technique is simple to practice, but it's also simple to binge on non-binge days. This is due to your brain's ability to deceive you into compensating for low-calorie days. Act as if your fasting never happened, as in the Eat Stop Eat model, to solve this dilemma.

Start the model by preparing your meals and gradually introducing the diet. Try not to make drastic dietary changes, as this will require too much willpower and can lead to burnout, causing you to revert to your old bad habits (or worse).

Fasting in this manner is a little rare. This fasting model allows you to eat whatever you want before going on a 36-hour fast.

The Fundamentals

You can eat whatever food you want with the Fast/Feast model, whether it's safe or unhealthy. You will lose weight quickly if you refrain from eating for an extended period of time. In addition, the diet can make it very simple to control your food cravings. The rules are as follows: you start with a complete cheat day, eating whatever you want, and then you fast for 36 hours. After that 36-hour fast, you'll have another complete cheat day followed by another 36-hour fast.

FAST/FEAST MODEL ADVANTAGES

Weight loss

Fasting for 36 hours reduces the amount of calories you consume. This will cause you to lose weight quickly.

Cheat Days in Full Swing

You can use the Fast/Feast Model to have absolute cheat days. This is great for satisfying a sweet tooth while still keeping the metabolism active.

It becomes easier to avoid unhealthy foods if cheat days are implemented. It will provide a mental and physical break for your body. You can prevent overeating fast food by removing food cravings.

Because of the following two factors, the approach is relatively difficult to follow:

1) It's very difficult to keep the calorie intake under control. Keeping track of calories on cheat days would be challenging for the majority of people. If you are unfamiliar with the calorie content of most foods, it is almost difficult to stay within your calorie cap.

2) Fasting for 36 hours can be very difficult. It can be difficult to maintain a 36-hour fast if you have never fasted before. The majority of people who do this version of Intermittent Fasting are already comfortable and experienced with it, which makes it easier for them to maintain.

Begin small with this model, as you did with the Alternate Day Diet. Instead of attempting a 36-hour fast all at once, start small by fasting for 12 hours and gradually raise the time.

How fasting affects the hormones:

1.   Hunger and fat storage hormones (leptin, insulin, + ghrelin)

Intermittent fasting takes center stage when it comes to reducing appetite, improving metabolism, and influencing blood sugar-related hormones. When patients have blood sugar issues, I prefer to prescribe intermittent fasting (IF) because it has been shown to improve metabolism and reduce insulin resistance. If you have a blood sugar problem and want to try fasting, it's important to consult with a doctor who can keep track of your progress and gradually increase your fasting time as your glucose levels stabilize. Leptin tolerance, another hormonal resistance pattern linked to weight gain and resistance to weight loss, has been shown to increase with IF.

And if you think fasting would make you hungry, you're mistaken. Intermittent fasting has been shown to have a beneficial impact on the appetite hormone ghrelin, which can increase brain dopamine levels directly (15). This is a great example of the gut-brain axis connection's truth.

The brain-ovary axis, also known as the hypothalamic-pituitary-gonadal (HPG) axis, connects your brain and ovaries. Your ovaries are signaled to release estrogen and progesterone by hormones released by your brain. If your HPG axis isn't functioning properly, it can affect your overall health and cause fertility issues.

Women are more receptive than men when it comes to intermittent fasting. This is because women have more kisspeptin, which makes them more responsive to fasting. If not done correctly, IF may cause women's cycles to be disrupted and their hormones to be thrown off. Although more research is needed, it is reasonable to assume that this hormonal change may influence metabolism and fertility as well.

All of this is to suggest that, since everyone is different, intermittent fasting is not for everyone. It's possible that you'll have to take a different path.

Crescendo fasting is a good way to progressively incorporate fasting into your daily routine.

Fast twice a week on non-consecutive days (such as Sunday and Thursday).

On fasting days, just do light exercise.

Between 12 and 16 hours is a good time to fast.

Add one more day of fasting to your schedule after a minimum of two weeks.

Branched-chain amino-acid supplements (BCAAs), which come in powder and capsule form, should be added around 6 grams during this period. These will help to boost the benefits of fasting and take the edge off.

3. CORTISOL (ADRENAL HORMONE):

Your adrenal glands, which sit right on top of your kidneys, release cortisol, which is your body's key stress hormone. When the brain-adrenal (HPA) axis is disrupted, cortisol levels may become unbalanced. Adrenal exhaustion is the product of this high-low rollercoaster. I've discovered that people who have problems with their circadian rhythm have a hard time with intermittent fasting. However, if you have someone to track your progress, you may be able to try a slow beginner intermittent fasting protocol or crescendo fasting.

The thyroid gland is the queen of all hormones, influencing every cell in your body. That is a force that no other hormone possesses. Nothing else matters if the thyroid hormones aren't working properly. Thyroid disorders come in a variety of forms, each of which can be influenced by intermittent fasting in a different way. As a result, I suggest consulting with a functional medicine practitioner who is familiar with your particular health situation.

For women, intermittent fasting may be challenging.

With all of these advantages, you may be wondering why someone wouldn't give it a shot. I do recommend it to the majority of my clients – as long as they keep those factors in mind.

Weight loss is difficult for anyone, but it appears that intermittent fasting has caused significant problems for some women, including binge eating, a delay in menstrual cycles, metabolic abnormalities, and early-onset menopause, even in younger women. Although most of this research is anecdotal, I've learned enough to advise caution when beginning an intermittent fasting regimen. It's important to consult with a trusted healthcare provider before embarking on a fasting regimen. Every woman has her own set of conditions, some of which may make her body extremely sensitive to calorie restriction. Calorie restriction can cause lower metabolism, fatigue, loss of fertility, nutritional deficiencies, weaker bones, and an increased risk of infection or illness due to a weakened immune response in some women.

I'm not saying this to scare you, and I still think intermittent fasting will benefit the majority of women. However, it's important to be aware of the risks associated with any weight-loss program. What causes these negative consequences? Hormones are at the root of everything (as they are with so many other health issues, especially among women). If you've read most of my writing, you're aware that hormonal imbalances can have a negative impact on almost every aspect of one's health. That's why, no matter what your aspirations are, it's important to see hormone wellbeing as part of the bigger picture.

Low calorie intake can disrupt the development of gonadotropin-releasing hormone (GnRH), which helps the release of two reproductive hormones: luteinizing hormone (LH) and follicle stimulating hormone (FSH) (FSH). These hormones are supposed to communicate with the ovaries, and if they don't, irregular cycles, infertility, and other problems may result.

This breakdown of communication also affects estrogen and progesterone, which are essential for ovulation and a healthy pregnancy, among other things. So, what exactly does all of this imply? Should women completely stop intermittent fasting? My response is an emphatic NO. All you have to do now is listen to your body and figure out what would work best for you. If you experience signs of hormonal deficiency after beginning intermittent fasting, you can consult with your doctor to see if you can proceed.

Fasting can also be avoided by a few groups of people, including pregnant mothers, babies, and small children. People with eating disorders, Type 1 diabetes, anyone who is seriously underweight, extreme athletes, and people on certain types of drugs, particularly diabetes medication, anti-seizure medication, and corticosteroids, may want to do this with the aid of a qualified functional medicine practitioner.

Now that you know what intermittent fasting is, how it can improve your health, and the risks it poses, especially to women, I'd like to share some of my best tips for lowering those risks. There is no one-size-fits-all solution that will work for everyone, but with so many fasting choices available, I'm sure that most women will find one that will.

√ *Determine which fasting approach is best for you.*

Fasting for a shorter period of time (say, 12 hours instead of 16 hours) will help limit the hormonal effects of fasting. Other strategies that women use to achieve weight loss success without side effects include fasting on alternate days rather than a normal fasting regimen, or consuming a limited amount of calories (about 25% of usual intake) on fasting days.

√ *Avoid nutrient shortages that can lead to hormonal imbalances.*

Whatever weight-loss tool you use, it's important to ensure that your body gets the vitamins, minerals, and nutrients it needs. That's why it's crucial to consume balanced, whole foods during non-fasting times. Unfortunately, it isn't always sufficient. Because of farming practices and nutrient degradation, getting the right nutrients can be difficult at any time. That's why, whether my clients are dieting or not, I still prescribe a high-quality multivitamin. You may also need additional support for hormonal balance; consult with your healthcare provider to decide the best regimen for you.

It's not to suggest you shouldn't exercise at all; it's just that if your calorie intake is extremely poor, you won't have the stamina to do high-intensity aerobic workouts. Yoga, stretching, Pilates, and walking are all excellent ways to keep the body active without overworking it.

During your menstrual period, your hormones are already functioning overtime. Rather than putting more pressure on your body, it's best to respect it and the hard work it's already doing. Remember that calorie restriction puts a burden on your body and triggers the stress response as though you were in a true famine. Too much stress can cause long-term hormone imbalance issues as well as other serious issues.

You are the greatest judge of your own body, and you will know if anything doesn't feel right. Working with a trusted professional gives you access to expert guidance as well as the opportunity to easily find a new solution if the one you're using isn't working. Remember that in order to lose weight and keep it off, you must change both your attitude and your eating habits. That's why it's important to adjust the strategy in order to find long-term solutions.

Intermittent fasting can be a fantastic way to change your eating habits from excessive snacking and food obsession to only eating when you're actually hungry. Often, once you start fasting, you'll find that you've been eating for reasons other than hunger!

However, launching into a strict fasting regimen right away isn't the best solution. Begin by deciding when you will avoid eating in the evening. Make sure you eat a healthy dinner that will keep you satisfied until breakfast, and then don't eat anything else until breakfast. Slowly extend the duration of your fast by moving dinner or breakfast sooner or later. Another choice is to fast one day a week, whether that means eating nothing or eating a significantly reduced number of calories.

Instead of the standard Intermittent Fasting regimen, which could see you fasting anywhere from 12 to 20 hours a day, crescendo fasting reduces the time to only two to three non-consecutive days of the week. The term "crescendo fasting" accurately describes its goal: gradually increasing the amount of fasting your body can tolerate.

So, for example, you could fast for 14 hours, beginning at 9 p.m. on Sunday and ending at 11 a.m. on Monday. After that, you'll eat normally for the next few days before repeating the fast. It's straightforward and easy to obey. It also relieves a lot of stress if you have trouble doing Intermittent Fasting on a regular basis.

Additionally, your body will be able to adjust to longer fasts over time, allowing you to adopt a more conventional Intermittent fasting schedule.

If you're a woman, you've probably found that men have an easier time losing weight than women. For us girls, this can be aggravating! This necessitates heightened awareness of our bodies. Hormones play a big role in a woman's wellbeing, and when they're out of whack—due to things like stress or the way we eat—it can have a big impact on our energy levels, mood, and even how hungry or full we feel.

When we're trying to improve our bodies, we can go a little crazy with calorie restriction, fasting, and exercise, for example.

All of this results in a lot of unnecessary stress on our bodies. And the way our bodies react to stress is by increasing the release of some hormones that cause us to hang on to our fat or even store more of it.

Imbalanced hormones can make weight loss difficult, and if you're starving yourself every day through Intermittent fasting, you'll likely become exhausted and ravenous, eating whatever you can get your hands on. Your body will also begin to break down lean muscle for fuel rather than fat.

Crescendo fasting, on the other hand, works softly with hormones to maintain a healthy balance, allowing you to maintain your metabolism and energy while also losing body fat.

You'll still be fasting, but only for shorter periods of time and less often. This is a healthy way to reduce your calorie intake and start losing weight without putting your body in a stressful starvation mode.

After a while, you might feel more at ease fasting for longer and more regular periods of time.

To get you started on a crescendo fasting strategy, here's a quick guide with some simple rules:

- √ On different days of the week, you can fast. Fast for 2-3 days that are not consecutive. You would want to fast on Sundays, Tuesdays, and Fridays, for example.
- √ Try to fast for 12-16 hours at a time on these days. This isn't as difficult as you would imagine. This ensures that if you finish your meal at 9 p.m., you will eat your next meal as early as 9 a.m. or as late as 1 p.m. the next day.
- √ You may want to take BCAAs on days when you're fasting (branched chain amino acids). These will help your body develop new muscle tissue, reduce muscle damage, and speed up healing by satisfying your appetite, supporting protein synthesis, and assisting in the building of new muscle tissue, reducing muscle damage, and speeding up healing.
- √ Choose light exercise or yoga over a high-intensity workout on your fasting days as well.

√ On non-fasting days, save the more rigorous exercises, such as HIIT or strength training.

√ Always remember to remain hydrated, whether you're fasting or not. Of course, water is best, but you can also add tea or coffee, but these can dehydrate you on their own. Drink at least 64 ounces of water a day to make sure you're getting your electrolytes. (This is why high-quality electrolytes are so essential, particularly on a ketogenic diet.) If you're drinking something else, make sure it's free of added sugars or artificial sweeteners.

√ When you've finished fasting for the day, make sure to eat all of your macros for the rest of the day; you don't want to skimp on calories, and you'll need to help your body "break" the fast.

√ If you find that this approach is working for you after two weeks, you may want to add another day of fasting to your schedule

√ The most important thing to remember is to avoid being upset! The aim of crescendo fasting is to acclimate your body to fasting. This is a much more long-term and reliable method of Intermittent fasting, particularly for women.

Although not all women would have a negative reaction to traditional Intermittent fasting protocols, most will have more success with crescendo fasting—especially if this is your first time fasting.

Jumping straight into an IF plan on a regular basis can be too hard on your body, causing uncontrollable hunger pangs, mood swings, exhaustion, and possibly weight gain.

You're much less likely to develop some bad eating patterns when you're just fasting over 12-16 hours for 2-3 days. When women begin a strict IF diet, they sometimes consume too few calories. This would just slow your metabolism and reduce the amount of lean muscle you have. The trick is to gradually introduce intermittent fasting so that you can operate with rather than against your hormones. Women are more likely to benefit from 2-3 days of crescendo fasting per week rather than a hardcore IF schedule.

However, crescendo fasting, like IF, requires calorie restriction, which can lead to weight loss, increased energy, and even a lower risk of chronic diseases like type 2 diabetes and cardiovascular disease.

If you adopt a ketogenic diet, these advantages can be enhanced even more.

Crescendo fasting is a relatively recent phenomenon, so the scientific community will have to catch up. However, a large study on the effects of intermittent fasting on female rats may provide insight into how intermittent fasting can be harmful to women if performed too rapidly and vigorously. Rats fasted for a full day every other day for 12 weeks in this 2013 report. The researchers found that the females' hormones were totally out of control after just two weeks. Their periods ceased, their ovaries shrank, and they had more insomnia than their male counterparts. Although these are some startling findings, they don't reveal anything about the impact of IF in female humans. They followed a strict fasting regimen that most of us wouldn't be able to maintain.

Aside from animal experiments like this, nothing is known about how IF affects men and women differently. So, for the time being, we can only go on our own knowledge, and if you've noticed that intermittent fasting isn't working for you, we suggest attempting crescendo fasting.

One of the best aspects about the keto diet, as well as fasting, is that it forces you to pay attention to how the body reacts and is stimulated. You will begin to understand what factors influence your weight, mood, and energy levels, as well as what you can do to change any of these factors.

When can crescendo fasting be stopped?

Even though crescendo fasting is the gentlest form of fasting, it isn't for all. There may be something else going on in your body if your menstrual cycle is interrupted or you constantly feel exhausted and run-down. There's also the possibility that you're consuming too few calories. This may be the first symptom of an eating disorder, which you may or may not be aware of.

Fasting, particularly in younger women, can increase the risk of anorexia, binge eating, and bulimia. If you're experiencing these symptoms, it's best to break your fast and resume your daily eating schedule. If you think there's something else going on, you should see a doctor.

Is crescendo fasting right for you?

If you've been curious about intermittent fasting or have tried it and decided it's not for you, suggest a crescendo fasting strategy. Jumping straight into a regular Intermittent fasting schedule, particularly if you're a woman, can be dangerous to your health.

You might find that reducing your fasting times to 12-16 hours and your fasting days to only 2-3 days per week is much more beneficial—and sustainable. So that you can stick to your plan, choose particular days and times that fit best for you and your schedule. The main goal of crescendo fasting is to become more in tune with your body. You'll be able to automatically cut out a significant number of calories as a result of this procedure, which will aid weight loss.

Over time, you'll notice some of the other advantages associated with intermittent fasting, such as increased stamina, a healthier mind, and, for women, a balanced hormonal balance.

Your body will finally adjust to this fasting lifestyle and be able to handle more of it. If it continues to support you and your health goals, you will find that you will progress to a full-fledged intermittent fasting schedule. And, if you're starting a keto diet and want to improve your ketones and lose weight, crescendo fasting is a great way to get started.

CHAPTER 4: BENEFITS OF INTERMITTENT FASTING FOR WOMEN OVER 50

You've probably heard that eating a well-balanced diet is important. As a result, it's strange to believe that depriving yourself of a meal or more may be a requirement. Surprisingly, evidence suggests that intermittent fasting has health benefits. Intermittent fasting in various ways will have additional benefits in addition to weight loss. Intermittent fasting has a number of advantages, including:

Loss of weight and body fat

The majority of people who experiment with intermittent fasting do so in order to lose weight. Unlike other weight-loss methods, intermittent fasting forces you to adhere to a strict eating schedule that dictates when you should eat and when you should fast. The concept behind intermittent fasting is that it allows you to be more flexible while still requiring you to consume less meals. This is not the same as calorie counting, which is common in most weight-loss programs. When you change your dietary habits, you're more likely to eat less and consume less calories.

In addition, intermittent fasting improves hormonal function, which aids weight loss. That is, a decrease in insulin levels, combined with a higher presence of growth hormone and a rise in the amount of norepinephrine, accelerates the breakdown of fat into energy. As a result, fasting for a short period of time will boost your metabolic rate, allowing you to burn more fat. As a result, intermittent fasting helps you lose weight by lowering your calorie intake and increasing your metabolic rate. Intermittent fasting is thought to help you lose up to 8% of your body weight in 3 to 24 weeks. When you lose a lot of weight, your waist circumference shrinks as well, meaning that you're losing dangerous belly fat.

√ **Glucose levels remain stable**

Intermittent fasting will improve the way your body responds to sugar, according to studies performed on both humans and mice. Researchers were able to revert diabetes in mice by rebooting the pancreas that produces insulin. Individuals with high blood sugar have been shown to benefit from various types of fasting that include prolonged hours of unrestricted eating accompanied by five days of eating a limited fasting diet.

√ **Type 2 diabetes can be averted by losing weight, eating a balanced diet, and getting more exercise.**

If you lose weight, your insulin sensitivity increases, lowering your blood sugar. When you feed, the body releases insulin into your bloodstream, which provides energy to your cells. If you're pre-diabetic, though, you're insulin resistant, which means your blood sugar levels are consistently high.

According to science, intermittent fasting may help regulate glucose levels by forcing the body to produce insulin less frequently, restoring insulin secretion and encouraging new insulin-producing pancreatic beta cells.

√ **Improves the stability of the digestive system.**

The cells of the gastrointestinal tract are still busy. These cells may work to the point of being passed out as excreta in some cases. By ensuring that your body enters autophagy, you can restore these digestive cells with intermittent fasting. This eliminates the old cells and stimulates the immune system in the process. This is also true of a chronic autoimmune reaction that can cause bowel inflammation. Allowing them to rest helps them to restore and rebuild themselves.

Autophagy and an extended night fast will allow your gut to not only relax but also recharge.

√ **Better mental wellbeing**

Intermittent fasting has been shown in mice studies to enhance brain health by increasing mental performance. The amount of blood flowing to your brain decreases as you get older, while neurons shrink and brain volume decreases. Intermittent fasting slows down the aging process and keeps you mentally fit.

Intermittent fasting will help you avoid neurodegenerative disorders like Parkinson's and Alzheimer's by improving your brain health. Fasting also helps you lose weight and protects you from diabetes, which can increase the risk of Alzheimer's disease. Intermittent fasting also helps to improve the brain by preventing nerve cell degeneration. Intermittent fasting, according to one report, is critical in protecting neurons in the brain from excitotoxic stress. It also helps the body kill damaged cells while creating new ones by speeding up autophagy in neurons. This is critical in aiding the body's defense against disease. Intermittent fasting also improves the memory and learning capacity. Memory and mood have been shown to improve after periods of calorie restriction in studies.

√ **Cancer incidence is reduced.**

Over the last few years, cancer has become more common, affecting people of all ages and races. The good news is that autophagy has the potential to reduce the risk of cancer. Medical professionals are interested in autophagy because of its function in cancer prevention. Since cancer is caused by a cellular disorder, it helps to prevent cancer by encouraging cell inflammation, regulating the damage response to DNA by foreign bodies, and regulating genome instability.

√ **Longevity is promoted.**

Intermittent fasting has been shown to help people live longer lives. This idea dates back to the 1950s, when scientists discovered autophagy and realized how important it could be in deciding life quality. To put it another way, you don't need to consume a lot of nutrients to stay healthy; instead, focus on supporting the internal mechanism that recycles damaged cell parts and removes harmful body cells.

√ **Boost the immune system.**

When it comes to keeping your immune system in top shape, autophagy is powerful and reliable. It accomplishes this by inducing cell inflammation and actively fighting diseases through non-selective autophagy. As the immune system is attacked by pathogens, cellular inflammation strengthens the immune system's cells. By depriving cell proteins of nutrients, autophagy causes them to function more effectively, inducing inflammation. This triggers the immune response needed to keep diseases and infections at bay. It also removes dangerous elements from the cell, such as tuberculosis, microbacterium, and other essential components.

√ **Inflammation is regulated.**

Depending on the situation, autophagy may either minimize or improve the immune response. As a result, inflammation is both prevented and promoted. Autophagy increases inflammation by signaling the immune system to attack when there is a harmful invasion. It can, on the other hand, reduce inflammation within the immune system by removing the signals that cause it.

√ **A higher standard of living**

There are a plethora of tools and approaches available on the internet to ensure good health and a good life in general. The reality is that none of these approaches, which include diets, anti-aging creams, and other items, can help you get closer to autophagy during intermittent fasting. The cellular degeneration and regeneration processes that occur during autophagy will make you look younger than your actual age. This is particularly important for skin that has been exposed to harsh elements such as pollution and other chemicals that cause wrinkles, resulting in a decrease in skin quality with toxic substances forming layers over your skin cells.

√ **Neurodegenerative disease risk is reduced.**

You'll have a lower chance of developing neurodegenerative disorders like Alzheimer's and Parkinson's if the body achieves autophagy. Here's how to do it. The accumulation of toxic and old neurons in certain parts of the brain will cause neurodegenerative diseases to spread to the surrounding areas. As a result, autophagy effectively keeps these diseases in check by replacing the neuron sections that are no longer useful and replacing them with new ones.

√ **Mental efficiency is improved.**

Intermittent fasting improves cognitive performance while also increasing brain capacity. Intermittent fasting increases the rate of brain-derived neurotrophic factor (BDNF). This is a protein found in the brain that interacts with the parts of the brain that regulate learning, memory, and cognitive functions.

The neurotrophic factor derived from the brain can also defend and stimulate the development of new brain cells. When you fast intermittently, the body enters a ketogenic state, where ketones are used to convert body fat to energy. Ketones can also feed your brain, resulting in increased mental productivity, stamina, and comprehension.

√ **Disease prevention is essential.**

Intermittent fasting has been linked to disease prevention. Intermittent fasting, according to studies, improves a variety of risk markers for cardiovascular disease, including lowered cholesterol, lower blood pressure, and decreased insulin resistance. According to a study published in the World Journal of Diabetes, patients with type 2 diabetes who practice short-term regular intermittent fasting lose weight and have higher post-meal glucose variability. Intermittent fasting also improves stress tolerance, lowers inflammation and blood pressure, and improves glucose circulation and lipid levels, both of which lower the risk of cardiovascular diseases like cancer, Alzheimer's, and Parkinson's. By raising the levels of tumor-infiltrating lymphocytes, Intermittent fasting can also delay the development of some cancers including skin and breast cancer. These are the cells that the immune system sends to battle the tumor.

√   **Physical health has improved.**

Intermittent fasting has an effect on your digestive system and, as a result, your physical fitness. Food digestion is aided by having a short feasting window and a long fasting window. As a result, you consume a balanced and equal amount of food and calories on a daily basis. It's doubtful that you'll feel hungry once you've gotten used to this procedure. You won't have to worry about your metabolism slowing down because intermittent fasting will actually improve it, making it more flexible because your body will be able to run on both fats and glucose for energy. The use of oxygen is critical to your training's success. In reality, you must change your breathing patterns during workouts in order to perform well. The maximum amount of oxygen used by your body per kilogram of body weight or per minute is referred to as VO2. This is often referred to as wind. Your output is influenced by the amount of wind.

More wind equals greater comprehension. As a result, top athletes will have double the VO2 level of those who do not exercise. The VO2 levels of both the fasted and non-fasted groups were 3.5L/min at the start of the analysis, which was conducted on a fasted group who missed breakfast and a non-fasted group who had breakfast an hour before. The fasting group's wind increased by 9.7%, while those who ate breakfast saw a 2.5 percent increase.

√   **It improves bodybuilding.**

When you have a limited feasting window, you can eat less meals per day, allowing you to concentrate your daily calorie intake into 1-2 meals. This method is superior to dividing your calories into 5-6 meals during the day, according to bodybuilders. Maintaining muscle mass necessitates a certain amount of protein. Even though intermittent fasting does not concentrate on protein intake, you can maintain muscle mass with this eating pattern. You will keep your muscles even though you don't eat proteins or drink protein shakes and bars because your growth hormone hits incredible levels after 48 hours of fasting.

√   **Insulin sensitivity has improved.**

Insulin sensitivity refers to the level of sensitivity of the body cells in response to insulin. Insulin sensitivity that is high is beneficial. It helps your cells to use blood glucose more efficiently, lowering the amount of sugar in your system. Insulin resistance occurs when the insulin levels are too low. If this occurs, you'll have abnormal blood sugar levels, which, if not treated, will lead to type 2 diabetes. Insulin sensitivity varies from person to person and can change due to dietary conditions and lifestyle choices. As a result, enhancing it could be helpful to those who have type 2 diabetes or are at risk of developing it.

Intermittent fasting can reduce insulin resistance, according to a 2014 study of the effects of intermittent fasting in obese and overweight adults. Even so, there was no discernible difference in glucose levels. When achieved correctly, Intermittent fasting yields excellent results. Intermittent fasting has a number of advantages, ranging from weight loss to type 2 diabetes reversal. Even so, in order to see results, you must remain committed to and compliant with the intermittent fasting regimen.

Most importantly, make sure you set a target for yourself at the start of your fasting time. While you're at it, keep in mind that, unlike many weight-loss diets, fasting doesn't have a set length because it's just about depriving the body of food for a period of time. Instead of being strange or queer, Intermittent fasting is just a part of daily life. It's the most successful and oldest intervention you can imagine. And, despite its ability to rejuvenate the body and its healing potential, many people are unaware of it. If your aim is to lose weight, you don't have to place any pressure on yourself to achieve results right away. Take your time transitioning and allowing your body to adapt. This could mean beginning with a diet that is similar to your current one and gradually progressing to intermittent diets that enable you to fast for longer periods of time.

There is no way to succeed in a lifestyle change program unless you set a target for yourself. Achievable milestones will act as path markers for the rest of the lifestyle change journey.

Achievable milestones will act as path markers for the rest of the lifestyle change journey.

You're like a driver who gets in the car and starts driving without knowing where he or she is going if you don't have these guides. However, before you can find out how to set your goals, you must first conduct an objective self-assessment.

This method will strengthen your determination and assist you in sticking to your intermittent fasting plan. With that knowledge, you can summon the courage to keep moving forward and tackle the inevitable roadblocks that life throws our way.

Knowing your current weight and body shape is also invaluable knowledge. Knowing where you are when you begin will help you keep track of your progress when you integrate intermittent fasting into your daily routine. This chapter focuses on determining where you are now and where you want to be in the future (your long-term health and wellness goals).

Fasting tracker for life

Your weight history and a fearless self-inventory will help you get to the bottom of your bulge issue. With this knowledge, you can see past events and understand the impact food has had on your life. If awareness is strength, then getting a better understanding of yourself will help you gain control of your eating habits. The self-questions inventory's will also help you understand that while you can't change past, you can equip and improve yourself for the future. Examine your previous attempts, struggles, and weight-loss results with a critical eye. When complacency sets in, defining why you want to lose weight will help you stay motivated.

Ask yourself these questions when placing yourself under a microscope. Write down your thoughts in a journal or notebook.

» *Were you overweight when you were a kid? If that's the case, how did your parents react?*

» *Is your weight affecting your self-confidence? If so, explain how.*

» *Is your weight or the number on the scale affecting your mood? If so, explain how.*

» *Is your weight having an effect on your relationships? If so, explain how.*

» *When you're stressed, do you turn to comfort food? If so, describe how and when.*

» Is it true that fitting into clothes or not fitting into them has an effect on your mood? If so, explain how.

» How many diets have you attempted over the course of your life? Describe them in detail.

»Were you able to maintain your weight loss in the past? If so, how can you go about doing it?

» What would if you lost weight in the past and then gained it back?

» What causes you to overeat or binge eat, and what time of day does it happen? What is the lowest weight you have ever maintained as an adult for more than a few months? What were the circumstances of the incident?

» When was the last time you were at a weight you were comfortable with as an adult? What was your level of activity? » What were the conditions at the time? Have you ever had a doctor show concern about your weight? If you answered yes, explain your conversation with her.

This inventory will assist you in being motivated to make positive changes in your life. I recommend that you go through your answers again and again during your intermittent fasting journey. Reading your weight-related life history can be a strong motivator to get you back on track if you hit a snag in your new lifestyle.

Following a low-calorie, balanced diet and exercise schedule will undoubtedly assist you in losing weight. In any case, determining what motivates you to lose weight will aid you in your efforts to maintain your weight loss. Being mindful of the basic reason you need to get in shape promotes your success in achieving your goals and serves as an excellent catalyst for pursuing and maintaining your goals.

Here are a few of the most commonly accepted explanations why people need to lose weight. Sort through the following to see which ones inspire you the most:

» **Maintaining good health**: Being overweight is bad for your health because it increases circulatory strain (the silent executioner) and increases the risk of cardiovascular disease, diabetes, and specific diseases (such as bosom malignant growth). Keeping these illnesses at bay can be a big help for people who want to get in better shape. Maintaining a consistent way of life allows you to live a longer and higher-quality life.

» **Increasing your energy level**: It can sound counterintuitive, but intermittent fasting actually increases your energy level. Extra body fat takes energy to maintain, so losing it allows you to focus more of that energy on living your life.

» **Feeling better about oneself**: Obesity is stigmatized by society, which sends out messages that slim is in and fat is out. People's self-esteem will suffer as a result of this very real social shaming. Self-confidence can be harmed by embarrassment regarding one's appearance, which can lead to anxiety and depression. The desire to improve one's self-esteem and appearance is a powerful motivator to lose weight.

» **Reducing joint problems**: Joint pain, especially in the knees, is a common side effect of being overweight. Too much bodyweight puts strain on the joints, which can lead to wear and tear and, in the worst-case scenario, arthritis. Joint pain can be excruciating, creating a vicious cycle that increases weight gain by limiting the opportunity to exercise.

When you decide to adopt a new way of life, you must change your habits. Shift in behavior necessitates dedication and practice, but most importantly, you must understand how to set goals that are realistic for you.

Setting goals is important for long-term behavior change. Every week, you should ideally set one small target. To improve your chances of success, your goals should: » Reflect concrete acts rather than wishful thinking; » Include your own personal interests and activities that you enjoy, which will increase your chances of success. Goals should be written in the form of SMART objectives.

These parts go further into what SMART goals are and how you can build your own.

What are smart targets, and how do you set them?

The following are the elements of a SMART goal:

» **Specific**: Rather than saying, "I want to follow the 16:8 intermittent fasting schedule," say, "I'll confine my eating window to a given eight-hour window every day for the next seven days."

» **Measurable**: You must be able to demonstrate that you met your objective. Instead of saying, "I'll pick what time I want to eat each day when it comes," say, "I'll mark off on the intermittent fasting program that I ate during my fixed fasting window every day."

» **Actionable**: The target should be action-oriented. "Every day, I'll eat between 12 and 8 p.m. and just consume calorie-free drinks throughout my fasting hours." The verbs eat and drink are action verbs.

» **Realistic**: Your target should be something you think you can accomplish, not something too difficult. Assume you know you can quickly stop eating or consuming calorie-containing foods from the moment you wake up until 1 p.m., and that you can continue fasting from 8 p.m. until noon the next day. In that case, you will achieve this aim.

» **Time-bound**: It's important to set a deadline for your target so that you know when it'll be completed. For most people, a week is a reasonable time period. If you're going to do the 16:8 intermittent fast, make a one-week schedule ahead of time — it'll keep you motivated because you'll have a deadline.

Shape your SMART target using the answers to the previous section's questions. For eg, "This week, I'll walk 20 minutes on my treadmill at a 20-minute per mile pace every day at 3 p.m. for the next seven days." Instead of "I want to start an exercise program," this is a SMART target. Take a look at how this objective is broken down:

» **Basic**: Treadmill walking for 20 minutes is specific.

» **Measurable**: You run on the treadmill for 20 minutes. Walking is an operation, so it's actionable.

» **Doable**: If you've previously walked for exercise, this strategy is doable.

» Walking for 20 minutes a day for the next seven days is time-bound.

Write the first weekly SMART target in a journal of your choosing, on a sheet of paper, or on your creative phone note pad. Make your target a tiny one that you know you'll achieve 100 percent of the time. You're not done until you've completed your first weekly SMART target. Do the following questions come to mind: » Did I meet my target this week? » If you answered yes, now is the time to make a new one. If not, determine the source of the problem and set a new, more attainable target.

You can set a big picture, long-term target in addition to your significant small, weekly SMART goal. Setting long-term targets, such as three months, will assist you in planning your intermittent fasting journey. Three months is like goldilocks: it's not too far away, but near enough to feel. Not only can the long-term target sheet include weight goals, but also health and wellness goals.

Here's an example of a reasonable three-month objective:

Weight: In the next three months, I'll lose ten pounds. To keep track of my success, I'll weigh myself on the scale.

Health: Losing this weight would help me lower my blood sugar (I'm pre-diabetic) and lower my diabetes risk. To keep track of this health indicator, I'll measure my fasting blood sugar.

Fitness: Losing weight and getting in shape would allow me to move more freely while hiking with my children. I'll put this to the test by completing the one-mile hike that I'm currently unable to complete.

Taking steps after you've achieved your objectives

It's not a big deal if you don't meet your weekly goal; simply create a new weekly SMART plan. Ascertain that this week's SMART target is more attainable. If you met your target, treat yourself to a simple pleasure such as a new book, a massage, or relaxing in a hot bath, whatever makes you happy. Have a huge party when you reach your long-term goals! You should write something meaningful in your calendar to reward yourself with, and then mark off the days and weeks as you get closer to that day.

Take note about what you're eating.

If you want to lose weight by intermittent fasting, you must first determine what your healthy weight range is. You can better understand your short-term (baby steps) and long-term (healthy weight range) goals with this detail (your finish line). The advantages of losing weight go beyond appearances. Getting to a healthier weight will help you avoid and treat risky health problems that can shorten your life. You also gain a boost of self-esteem, which is a valuable advantage. You may be satisfied with your current weight and just want to try intermittent fasting for the additional health benefits it provides, such as disease prevention and anti-aging effects. If you're thinking of trying intermittent fasting, talk to your doctor first. If you have been diagnosed with a chronic illness,

Intermittent fasting must be done under the supervision of your personal doctor.

Intermittent fasting is not permitted if you have an eating disorder. People come in all shapes and sizes, with a wide range of personal health and fitness experiences. Before determining what a healthy weight range is for you, you must first complete a few preliminary steps to help you determine what healthy weight range is appropriate for you.

Maintain your workout routine.

For most Americans, expanding abdominal girth and diminishing muscle mass are unavoidable side effects of aging. Participating in a daily workout routine is the most successful way to control and even avoid these symptoms. Although most people find exercising and intermittent fasting to be perfectly healthy, some people might not feel comfortable exercising while fasting. Now is not the time to start an intense fitness regimen if you haven't been exercising regularly. Before beginning any exercise program, always seek permission from your doctor or healthcare provider, particularly if you intend to combine exercise with an intermittent fasting plan.

CHAPTER 6: DEBUNKING THE COMMON MYTHS

With so much fitness and diet knowledge floating around the internet, it's easy to lose track of what's true and what's not. The advice on which diet to follow differs greatly; many are true, but there are also some popular misconceptions. People who are unaware that those myths are false may follow the wrong advice, sabotaging their own progress (despite having a strong work ethic). When I see anything like this, it makes me really angry. I used to be the newbie who would browse every forum on the internet, getting giddy at the prospect of putting the false advice I received into practice. And in the end, I'd sabotage my own advancement. Eventually, I realized that many of the misconceptions about nutrients and Intermittent Fasting were simply not true. But it wasn't until I met mentors who had the results, I desired that I realized exactly what I needed to do to achieve the same results.

To be frank, getting to the point that I could clearly see, and advice was false, and which wasn't took a long time and was extremely frustrating. I'd like to save you some time by dispelling some popular Intermittent Fasting myths. But first, allow me to clarify why and how myths are created:

1. **A lack of understanding and/or interest**

There are those who want to draw conclusions based on newly found scientific findings but lack the expertise to do so properly. They must first have an academic background in that area in order to better draw conclusions from the findings of a particular study. They don't have one most of the time, so they obviously draw false conclusions.

Aside from that, there are people who have the necessary expertise but keep saying the same thing over and over (while somewhat knowing that it is incorrect). This typically occurs when people lose interest in the area they're researching and don't want to put in the time and effort necessary to better interpret a particular finding.

Another major factor is scientists' fear of losing their reputation. When scientists discover that the opposite of what they teach is valid, it is extremely humiliating for them to admit that they were wrong about a particular topic. In order to maintain their reputation, scientists seldom report their newly discovered findings.

2. **The influence of others**

If you tell a lie enough times, it will finally become the truth. If you hear something that isn't (or isn't) true repeatedly, you'll finally believe it to be true. This is referred to as social conditioning. What is the reason for this? Since we don't have enough patience or resources as humans to try it out for ourselves. Others must "invent the wheel" for us so that we can concentrate on more important matters. As a result, while social conditioning can be extremely beneficial, it can also work against us. When these socially conditioned myths become widespread enough, it will be extremely difficult to debunk them and uncover the facts.

3. **Marketing (false)**

Supplement, food, and fitness companies are continually providing us with misleading details in order to sell us their goods. People who do not have enough information about fitness or nutrition profit immensely from these companies because they are easier to exploit. They deceive people who aren't well educated by manipulating and lying about their goods. The grain industry, for example, is constantly claiming that you should start your day with a nutritious cereal, and the food industry, which is constantly claiming that you should feed your body during the day, both profit from people who believe they need to buy vast amounts of food all of the time.

Myth #1: Intermittent fasting is linked to nutrient deficiency.

Many people believe that if you fast, you won't get enough vitamins, but this is not true. Fasting teaches the body to feed at regular intervals. You would not lose vital vitamins and/or minerals if you do this. Furthermore, the nutrients you lose during a fasting day are replenished when you feed. If you just want to drink your vitamins at specific times of the day, you can also take vitamin tablets.

Myth #2: To keep your blood sugar levels in check, you need to eat small meals during the day.

Small meals, according to some "food experts," will help you stabilize your blood sugar. However, when you are well, your blood sugar levels are well-controlled and managed. When you go without food for a few hours or even a day, they don't fluctuate as much.

Furthermore, from an evolutionary standpoint, going without food for a few hours, days, or even a week is perfectly natural. Our forefathers and mothers faced occasions when they didn't have access to food, but this didn't have a significant effect on their blood sugar levels. As a result, the myth that you must eat small meals during the day to keep your blood sugar levels in check is clearly untrue.

Myth #3: When you Fast, you will lose mostly muscle and very little fat.

In reality, the polar opposite is real. Fat is a high-energy molecule with several times the energy of protein (it is around 2 times more energy dense than protein). As a result, it makes sense for the body to use stored fats as an energy source before turning to protein. Furthermore, the primary function of fat is to provide us with energy when food is scarce. Since the proteins in our muscles produce much less energy, the body cannot efficiently use protein as an energy source. Furthermore, the main aim of protein is to ensure that our skeletal muscles and bodies work properly, rather than to provide energy to the body.

Furthermore, there is a significant difference between the calorie reserves contained in fats and proteins. Fat stores hold 85 percent of our calorie stocks, while protein stores hold 14 percent. Fat is, without a doubt, the most critical energy storage molecule. When food is scarce, our bodies make sense from a physiological perspective to turn to our fat stores for energy.

Myth #4: You're deliberately starving yourself.

We also mistakenly associate "missing those meals" with "starvation." We've become used to making food available to us at all times that we panic when we miss a meal. However, I would not consider missing a meal to be the same as starving yourself. True starvation occurs when your body's fat reserves are depleted and it starts to kill your muscles for energy, resulting in rapid death. This is not the case for Intermittent Fasting. Fasting times are brief, and you consume enough calories from your meals (in addition to fat reserves) to maintain your energy levels.

Myth #5: Skipping breakfast is bad for your health and will make you fat.

People who miss breakfast are more likely to be overweight. This is because most breakfast skippers have erratic eating habits and are unconcerned with their health. Another factor people who miss breakfast are heavier than those who don't is that they are more likely to be on a diet. Furthermore, being on a diet will result in binge eating. Dieters are often more likely to be overweight than non-dieters in the first place.

As a result, it's understandable that most people believe missing breakfast makes you fat. However, as previously said, it is what breakfast skippers do in addition to skipping breakfast that causes them to gain weight, not the fact that they skip breakfast.

Myth #6: Intermittent fasting has a negative impact on weight-lifting results.

Another myth that has been spread across the world without any true or credible evidence to back it up. Aerobic practices had an insignificant negative impact on the results of many people who were fasting during Ramadan, according to research. This is true even though you are dehydrated due to the fluid restrictions imposed by Ramadan.

Strength training is unaffected by fasting, except when the person is fasting for three days straight, according to more research that did not require the restriction of fluids. As a result, the idea that people can't perform well when fasting is completely false.

Myth #7: If you fast, you will be hungry.

The majority of people who first learn about Intermittent Fasting are afraid of going hungry while fasting. Although this might be valid at first when attempting to enforce Intermittent Fasting, it will certainly pass quickly. What is the reason for this? Almost everything we do in our daily lives is a product of habit formation. We develop behaviors so that our bodies don't have to rely on willpower to accomplish those tasks. However, when your body sends you a warning that you're hungry, it's really a habit cause. You are usually not hungry, but since you eat at that time every day, you will obtain a habit trigger.

It will be difficult to ignore these hunger causes when you first start Intermittent Fasting. This is due to the fact that it takes 30-60 days to develop a new habit or break an old one. If you stick with it for the first 60 days, you'll find it much easier to ignore these signals, and they might even go away. After that, the body can give hunger signals at various times during the day. So, for at least the first 60 days after you begin practicing Intermittent Fasting, ignore the hunger signals you get outside of your time windows. Your body can learn to give hunger signals at various times of the day if you do this correctly.

Intermittent fasting may be done in a variety of ways, but most experts suggest a 24-hour fast because it allows the body to cleanse itself without depriving it of the nutrients it needs. This is the most common and straightforward version, as it allows users to eat whatever they want while they are not fasting, but, as previously mentioned, the better you eat and the more intelligent your food choices, the faster you can lose weight.

Fasting for two 24-hour cycles over the course of a week could be the best solution. This is long enough to reap the benefits of fasting, but not so long that it becomes a chore to go without food every time.

If you fast for a 24-hour cycle once or twice a week, you'll be able to lose weight while still fasting the foods you like. Intermittent fasting works because it pays homage to the caveman period. It's now just a matter of figuring out if it's right for you. Intermittent fasting can be tried in a number of ways to see how it blends with your lifestyle.

Is it suitable for you?

Here are several ways to incorporate intermittent fasting into your daily routine.

Try a trial run.

√ Set aside a 24-hour cycle during which you will not consume any food. Start after dinner to make it easier, and take advantage of the time you'll be sleeping. The next day, miss breakfast and lunch and remain hydrated by drinking plenty of water and green tea.

√ Then eat a regular meal 24 hours after you last ate. Just be careful not to overeat. Otherwise, you'll eat the calories you saved by missing two meals.

√ This trial fast is also a perfect way to reset your body and get a healthy eating plan off to a good start. It helps your body to cleanse itself, giving you a clean slate to start with. What better time to start thinking of food as fuel and to start fueling your body with healthy stuff so that it can work hard for you?

√ Hold your waistline in control by fasting.
√ Daily fasting might be a perfect way to remain on track and lose weight for good if the test run went well and didn't result in a midnight attack on the refrigerator.

√ When you despise every minute of it, dietary adherence falls by the wayside. So, it's doubtful that you'll get back on the diet bandwagon after a failed grapefruit diet. Fasting for a few hours, on the other hand, takes less willpower and determination (after all, a meal is just a few hours away).

This version helps you to eat normally one day and fast the next. The program has the same positive health benefits as calorie restriction but without the negative mental and physical consequences. Experts devised an alternative day fast that encourages users to eat every day, making it easier to handle and ensuring that no day goes without food entirely.

The plan allows for a 24-hour fasting time, but since it begins at 6 p.m., no day is completely without food. Participants eat before 6 p.m. on the first day, which is a feeding day. Participants miss breakfast and lunch on the second day, consuming their next meal at 6 p.m. The next day is another feeding day, with days of fasting in between.

The benefit of this regimen was that we could eat every day. We'd have supper one day and breakfast and lunch the next. We will never go a day without eating.

The program is easier to follow because it eliminates the sense of deprivation that comes with a typical fast. This means that hunger pangs don't become so overwhelming that the fast ends with an entire pizza and a ride to your local drive-through for dessert.

This strategy is most similar to the caveman's, and it takes us much closer to the roots that our bodies still cling to. The three-square-meal-per-day routine has become ingrained in us as modern humans. Animals in the wild, particularly carnivorous animals, do not eat three times a day; instead, they eat when they kill something. I'm sure Paleolithic man did the same thing. If I had to make an educated guess, I'd say Paleolithic man ate once or twice every three days.

Many advocates of intermittent fasting believe that fasting on a regular basis – or minimizing the period during the day when food is permitted, known as an eating window – is the most effective way to lose weight and maintain a slim figure. Due to the limited time available to actually feed, decreasing the amount of mealtime automatically reduces calorie consumption!

Another advantage of eating this way is that you'll become more aware of the foods you consume. It's much more likely that your first meal after the fast will be meticulously prepared rather than a hasty all-you-can-eat binge.

A vital part of the 'transform' process is becoming more mindful of what you're eating. The war is almost won once you start making educated choices about the foods you consume based on whether they can provide you with energy and the nutrients you need rather than how they taste.

The trick to making the daily fast work for you is to make sure that the foods you eat before you begin your fasting period will properly fuel you during the fasting period, allowing you to power through your day without running out of energy.

Natural nocturnal fasting

Using the usual fast that comes with sleep means not eating after dinner – no midnight snacks or popcorn while watching TV – and continuing the fast in the morning. One way to make this fast work is to go to the gym before breakfast, which will put the body into fat-burning mode faster.

The earlier we quit eating in the evening, the longer the fast will last and the more benefits the body will reap. Internal energy is released as in any fasting process, which can then be used to cleanse and repair bodily tissues.

If you're interested in giving intermittent fasting a shot, try the week-long program below. It has two fasting times of 24 hours each. The majority of experts believe that it is the most efficient – and least intolerable – method of incorporating fasting into your life. Since most people choose to begin their diets at the beginning of the week, the program begins on Sunday evening, with the first fast taking place the next day, when you miss breakfast and lunch.

The first day

- Breakfast, lunch, and dinner are all available. Your first fast begins after dinner, so eat whatever you want today, concentrating on protein to keep you feeling fuller for longer. Consider eating more whole, unprocessed foods.

Eating as clean as possible – new fruits and vegetables, whole grains (think protein-rich quinoa, oatmeal, and brown rice), and proteins (chicken, Omega-3-rich salmon, beans, and lentils) – because these will fuel your body to perform at its best, and you'll feel stronger for it.

Protein has been shown to be the most satiating macronutrient of the lot, meaning it can hold you fuller for longer than carbohydrates or fat, gram for gram.

- Following dinner (6:30 p.m.) Your fast starts right now, but your body will not go into fasting mode until after midnight, when it has digested your Sunday evening meal.

Day 2 – 6:00 a.m. – 8:00 a.m. Congratulations, you've made it halfway through your first fasting cycle without even trying. If you regularly consume caffeine, drink a glass of water and a cup of coffee, and bring green tea and more water to work.

- 7 a.m. – Take your vitamins, which may include a multivitamin, a Vitamin D capsule, a tablespoon of fish oil or cod liver oil, and a branched-chain amino acid capsule, to help muscle repair and regeneration, before leaving the house.

- 12 o'clock Your fast is coming to an end. Continue to drink plenty of water and green tea, as well as a cup of hot coffee or tea to keep hunger at bay.

- 5:30 p.m. to 7:00 p.m. When you're on an intermittent fast, the safest time to exercise is when you're in fat-burning mode. Since it's crucial to refuel after your workout, this hour before you break your fast is ideal for hitting the gym, lacing up your running shoes, or getting on your bike.

Some experts recommend drinking a whey protein drink before working out to avoid working out on an empty stomach. However, you can tailor this to your personal preferences, as well as the type of workout you're doing. If you do cardio, you may feel a little sick, but if you do weights, you should be fine. It's best to try a few different things to see what works best for you.

– At 6:30 p.m. – It's time to break your fast now that you've gone 24 hours without eating. Be sure to include protein, fruits, and some fat in this first meal to get the most out of your workout. This meal should usually consist of 8 ounces of protein, as many vegetables as desired, a handful of nuts or seeds, and a serving of brown rice or another whole grain such as bulgar wheat, quinoa, or barley.

The third day is a non-fast day. Today, eat whatever you want, but keep in mind that rummaging through the refrigerator is not the best way to handle your body.

Continue to choose lean protein, and if you're planning a workout, add extra carbohydrates for more efficient energy. You want to boost your carbohydrate intake while lowering your fat intake on exercise days. On non-workout days, you can limit your carbohydrate intake while increasing your fat consumption.

Protein can stay reasonably stable from day to day, regardless of how fats and carbohydrates are manipulated.

The fourth day

- Breakfast, lunch, and dinner are all available. Your second fast begins after dinner today, so eat plenty of protein and fiber from vegetables and whole grains to stay satisfied.

Making smart food choices will help, and you'll notice that higher fat foods, such as fast-food meals, make you feel sluggish, while fresh foods give you energy and keep you feeling fuller for longer.

On the fifth day,

– 7:00 a.m. – You've made it halfway through your second fasting phase, and this time you know what to expect. Keep the same routine if you weren't hungry during your first fast. If you do get hungry, drink water laced with fiber supplements to make you feel better.

– 7:00 a.m. – Coffee and tea are good, but water is needed. A multivitamin, a Vitamin D capsule, a tablespoon of fish oil or cod liver oil, and a branched-chain amino acid capsule are all important supplements.

- 12 o'clock Drink plenty of water and green tea to stay hydrated. Staying hydrated also aids in the reduction of hunger.

- 5:30 p.m. – Use whey powder to fuel your workout and get to work on your favorite task.

- Break your fast at 6:30 p.m. Between now and bedtime, some experts recommend eating one or two meals. See what works best for you; don't just eat for the sake of eating; and remember that mindless or binge eating is not part of the plan.

Sixth day

- Today is not a fast day. Feel free to eat whatever you want today, just try to avoid eating too much fast food. Eating a protein-rich, well-balanced diet will give you much better results.

Seventh day

- Today is a day off. Today, disregard your self-imposed restrictions and eat whatever you want. Go out to a pub, order a bottle of wine (or two), and order dessert.

Knowing that you should indulge in your favorite foods on occasion makes every diet plan easier to stick to. After a few weeks of learning how foods affect you, you'll be more likely to make better decisions, even on your free days, such as choosing broiled over fried or poached over grilled, simply because you know which will make you feel sluggish and slow.

How To make it work for you

It's important to take intermittent fasting seriously if you're serious about trying it. It's a waste of time to fast for 24 hours and then eat junk food or eat half of your child's birthday cake because you didn't get a chance to eat it the day before because you were fasting.

With intermittent fasting, it's maybe more crucial than ever to make sure you're getting the right foods when you eat because your body has everything it needs to function without sending you into binge mode during the times you don't. On rest days, make protein the most important macronutrient. "On exercise days, make sure you eat some carbohydrates afterward and try to consume the rest of your calories afterward. Eat a lot of fruits and vegetables, as your mother always says.

The consistency of your food will have the greatest impact on whether or not intermittent fasting will work for you. The focus should remain on high-quality foods. Vitamins, minerals, and other essential nutrients found in whole natural foods are what your body needs. Slowly introduce IF into your diet, focusing on the quality of your foods, and you'll see results.

I'll teach you how to correctly execute Intermittent Fasting in this chapter. I recall making some crucial errors when I first began, which slowed down the process of introducing Intermittent Fasting. I'm going to teach you how to do Intermittent Fasting effectively and without making any mistakes.

Step 1: Begin with why.

You should understand the reasons behind everything you do in life. You will ultimately fail if you do those things without understanding why you are doing them. Intermittent Fasting is the same way. Before you begin, you must first determine why you want to implement Intermittent Fasting.

Our Individual Characteristics So, how do you go about doing this? Humans have a variety of traits (or different selves). There is a lower, a regular, and a higher self in each of us. Depending on the time, location, circumstance, and atmosphere, we appear to switch between these personalities during the day. - of these personalities is driven by something different, and you must bring them all together to achieve the same goal: introducing Intermittent Fasting. You will ultimately sabotage yourself if your target is not balanced between these personalities. As a result, the trick is to come up with motives for all of your identities to accomplish a specific objective that are emotionally convincing to you.

Let's say you're in a normal mood and unexpectedly decide to lose 10 pounds of body fat because you want to look better. You decide to go on a diet after realizing that you need to improve your eating habits. Going on a diet is a healthy thing to do, and losing body fat for the sake of "looking good" is a good excuse to do so. But there's a catch... you just know why your normal self needs to lose 10 pounds of body fat. What about your higher or lower self, though? What motivates 'them' to lose weight? What if you're in a stressed-out mood and want to eat fast food? You'll probably say to yourself, "Screw this diet," and sabotage yourself. Or, if you're in a higher self, you don't worry about appearances and say to yourself, "Why bother?"

How do we recognize our various personalities?

So, once again, the trick is to come up with explanations for all of your identities that are emotionally convincing to you. And how do you distinguish between your various personalities? Easy, based on your thinking patterns. When you have negative thinking patterns, you typically find yourself in your lower self. You are in your standard self when you have neutral feelings, and you are in your higher self when you have really positive thoughts.

Your Lower Self is guided by selfish, unreasonable, and slightly childish motivations such as being better than others, teaching others a lesson, being lazy, escaping responsibility, and so on.

Your Standard Self is driven by logical, rational, and ethical reasons such as understanding that you must do XYZ in order to achieve a specific outcome, remembering your duty, and so on.

Your Higher Self is guided by a higher meaning, such as empowering and encouraging others, making a positive impact on the environment, contributing to society, and so on.

Determine your own reasons for implementing intermittent fasting as an exercise.

It's time to decide your own reasons for implementing Intermittent Fasting now that you know how to build them. Take 10 to 30 minutes to sit down and write down all of the reasons why you want/need to start Intermittent Fasting. I've shown you all of the advantages of intermittent fasting, as well as how the most common misconceptions about it are clearly untrue. Take a moment to consider the factors that motivate you the most.

Make up additional personal explanations for implementing Intermittent Fasting. These arguments must be emotionally persuasive to you and should propel you closer to your target. It is also insufficient to provide only negative or optimistic motives for introducing Intermittent Fasting. Both are needed (and even logical reasons). Again, spend 10 to 30 minutes coming up with excuses for your lower, normal, and higher selves. Be sure to think of as many excuses as you can!

Note: Not to be pessimistic, but I already know that only a small percentage of people who are reading this book have completed the exercise. That's something I appreciate. I really dislike having to put down a book in order to complete an exercise. If you're serious about starting Intermittent Fasting, you can go back and complete the workout (if you haven't already). If you want to try Intermittent Fasting, this is a must-do move. I can already tell you that if you don't figure out why you want to do it, you're setting yourself up for failure.

Step 2: Decide which form of Intermittent Fasting you'd like to try.

In Chapter 2, I went over a few different Intermittent Fasting Models that you can use. These models are very similar, but the implementation differs. Again, the model you choose is entirely up to you, but it is dependent on your objectives. You should clearly identify your objectives and determine which Intermittent Fasting model is best for you.

Of course, the principles of these Intermittent Fasting models can be combined. I've used a combination of the Leangains and the Alternate Day Diet models, for example. I like the idea of the Leangains model, but some of the details aren't feasible for me. As a result, I wanted to make minor changes to the model by combining it with the Alternate Day Diet model.

To be truthful, if you're new to Intermittent Fasting, I wouldn't suggest creating a modification of the templates. I suggest that you first select a model, run it, and observe the results. If you notice that it isn't working for you, it may be a good idea to make some minor changes or try a different style.

Step #3: Break Down Your Selected Model's Principles Into Actionable Habits

All we do in life is, once again, a learned habit. Habits can be our most valuable asset or our most dangerous liability. Someone who exercises every day, for example, has developed a wonderful habit (read: asset). However, anyone who consumes fast food on a daily basis has developed a worrying habit (read: liability). You want to develop good habits that will help you achieve your objectives.

You want to develop good habits that will help you achieve your objectives. However, putting these behaviors into practice can be challenging because it takes a lot of willpower to form a habit. As a result, you'll want to break down all of the values into small routines that you can quickly enforce. It might seem like you aren't making any progress at first, but I assure you that you will if you stick with it. Often, avoid the trap of attempting to adopt too many patterns at once. You only have so much willpower, and implementing so many routines will fast deplete it, causing you to sabotage your progress or abandon the Intermittent Fasting model altogether.

To make it simpler for you, I've broken down all of the Intermittent Fasting models from Chapter 2 into small habits:

Leangains

Habit 1: Begin your eating window at X o'clock (the time you want to begin your eating window each day).

Habit 2: Break your eating window at X+8 hours (8 hours after you first started eating).

3A (For those who are trying to lose weight): Consume 25% of the total daily calorie intake in carbohydrates, 40% in protein, and 35% in fat.

Habit 3B (For people looking to gain weight): Make up half of your daily calories from carbohydrates, 35 percent from protein, and 15 percent from fat.

To gain weight properly, consume approximately 200-400 calories more than seen.

Habit 1: Begin your eating window at X hour (the time you want your eating window to begin each day, but it must be at night).

Habit 2: Break your eating window at X+4 hours (4 hours after you first started eating).

Habit 3: Replace unhealthy snacks (processed foods, for example) with fruits.

Habit 4: Outside of your eating window, start eating small portions of protein (around 100 calories per meal).

Replace bad drinks (soft drinks, for example) with fruit juice and water.

Eat stop eat

Habit 1: Pick a day for a 24-hour fast and begin by fasting for 12 hours on that day.

Habit 2: On that day, extend your fast to 16 hours.

Habit 3: On that day, extend your fast to 20 hours.

Habit 4: On that day, extend your fast to 24 hours.

Habit 5 (for those who want to fast for 24 hours on a different day): Repeat habits 1 through 4 on a different day.

Habit 1: Make sure you eat enough calories to maintain your weight on a daily basis.

Habit 2: On low-calorie days, eat 80% of your calories.

Habit 3: On low-calorie days, reduce this to 60% of your total calories.

Habit 4: On low-calorie days, reduce this to 40% of your total calories.

Habit 5: On low-calorie days, reduce this to 20% of your total calories.

Model of fasting and feasting

Habit 1: Fast for 12 hours and then eat normally for the rest of the day.

Habit 2: Fast for 18 hours and then eat normally for the rest of the day.

Habit 3: Observe a 24-hour fast with a regular day of eating.

Habit 4: Pursue a 32-hour fast with a cheat day.

Habit 5: Pursue a 36-hour fast with a cheat day.

Step #4: Re-evaluate and visualize your habits, then put one into action each month.

To better adopt the behaviors selected in step 3, you must do so gradually. Many people I know want to make a drastic change right away, so they plan to overhaul their diet in a week. This isn't the way to go about it! Every human being, no matter how strong their willpower, has a breaking point. The breaking point is when you've used all of your willpower and abandoned all of your chosen routines. When this happens, you are not progressing, and even worse, you are regressing!

So, how do you develop habits without exhausting your willpower? One habit per month should be implemented. Decide, for example, to start habit 1 on day 1 and keep it going until day 30. If you've completed habit 1 successfully, you can move on to habit 2. If you find yourself falling behind on habit 1 between days 1 and 30, restart the loop. I understand that it sounds tedious and inconvenient, but it is the only way to do it effectively. Also, keep in mind that the more you do something, the less difficult it becomes. The first week or two will be the most difficult, but after that, you can almost guarantee that you can complete the task.

Another thing to remember is that if you successfully followed the first habit but fail to do so when attempting to adopt habit 2, you can go back and start the 30 days over with habit 1. The aim isn't to do each habit for 30 days at a time, but to keep them going. As a result, always double-check that the earlier patterns are being followed when performing the newer ones.

Examine and visualize the routines

You should also set aside 10 minutes per day to study and imagine yourself carrying out the behaviors. You will continually remind yourself why you are doing what you are doing if you do this, and you will assist yourself in making the habit a reality. Read the reasons why you want to adopt such habits to effectively review your habit. After that, spend 7-10 minutes visualizing yourself effectively completing the habit.

"However, this is taking much too long!"

"Will it really take me 30 days to implement one tiny habit?" people ask me all the time. This means that I won't be able to completely enforce Intermittent Fasting for at least another 5-6 months! That was just too long!" On one hand, I understand their concern; 5-6 months is a significant amount of time. But, on the other hand, I'm not sure why they become discouraged. Isn't it wonderful to know that if you just take one little step forward every day, you'll achieve your goals?

When I was bad, I had one mindset: "I can either work hard and consistently for my goals and actually reach them, or I can do two things." Or I can whine and become discouraged by the amount of effort required to be effective, resulting in failure!" So, what exactly are you looking for?

One misconception I'd like to dispel is the notion that everyone learns at the same rate. This isn't correct. All progresses at their own pace. I've broken down the concepts of the Intermittent Fasting models into small routines, but that doesn't mean you won't be able to adopt one faster than I did. In reality, I know a lot of people who have completed it far more quickly. Those individuals, on the other hand, are fast learners. They can easily implement and learn new information. I am not one of those people, which is why I demonstrated the slowest method of implementing Intermittent Fasting.

If you are certain that you can do it quicker, please do so... However, if you are someone who is prone to procrastination, please take it slowly. Although the process will take longer, you will be able to keep up with it!

Note: If you find yourself struggling repeatedly after doing everything I've suggested, choose to break the patterns down into even smaller chunks. If you're a late learner, don't give up. The majority of my clients who are slow learners, even more so than fast learners, are the most good at what they do.

1. Beans

Fixings

- 1 pound (or 1/2 kilogram) of your #1 beans
- 1/2 pound (1/4 kilogram) hamburger or pork bones
- 2 narrows leaves
- 1 onion, diced
- 2 tablespoons olive oil or margarine
- 1 teaspoon ocean salt
- 1 teaspoon pepper

Headings

√ Clean and cover beans with water for the time being.

√ Simmer beans with bones and narrows leaves somewhere in the range of 2 and 4 hours on low warmth and covered. Pinto and bruised eye peas mellow rapidly while different beans, for example, kidney beans take longer.

√ Add the leftover fixings in the last half hour of cooking.

√ The way to great beans is the bones and oil. These two fixings make the beans heavenly. We don't hesitate to add extra flavors however we would prefer.

2. Bone Broth

Fixings

- 1/2 pound (1/4 kilogram) meat, chicken, fish, or pork bones
- 2 sound leaves
- 1 teaspoon ocean salt
- 1 teaspoon pepper

Bearings

√ Simmer bones and sound leaves in any event 3 hours on low warmth, covered.

√ Add the salt and pepper in the last half hour of cooking.

3. Carrot and Cucumber Salad

Fixings

- 1 carrot
- 1 enormous cucumber
- 2 tablespoons rice or white vinegar
- 2 tablespoons nectar
- 1 teaspoon ocean salt
- 1 teaspoon pepper

Headings

√ Clean both the carrot and cucumber. Cut the cucumber the long way and utilize a spoon to eliminate the seed center. Julienne both the carrots and cucumbers. We may change the quantity of carrots and cucumbers to get a proportion of coordinated.

√ Julienne, a unique shredder from the Asian stores, shreds vegetables into long shoestrings.

√ Mix all fixings together.

√ Malaysians offer varieties of this dish. Now and then, they dice and add pineapple or diced zesty chilies.

Carrot Salad

Fixings

- 3 carrots
- 1/4 cup white vinegar or apple juice vinegar
- 1/4 cup water
- 2 tablespoons nectar
- 1/2 teaspoon ocean salt
- 1/2 teaspoon dark or white pepper
- 3 cloves, finely diced garlic
- 3 shallots finely diced or 1/2 red onion finely diced

Headings

√ Mix the vinegar, water, nectar, salt, pepper, shallots, and garlic together. Permit the sauce to assimilate the flavors.

√ Julienne the carrots. Julienne is an extraordinary shredder, for the most part at Asian stores, that shreds vegetables into long shoestrings.

√ Bring a pot of water to bubble. Add the carrots and whiten for 10 seconds. Indeed, 10 seconds. Strain carrots and flush with cold water. Whiten mollifies the carrots a touch.

√ Drizzle olive oil and sauce and refrigerate for an hour to permit carrots to retain the flavors.

√ The venders make a zesty adaptation of this serving of mixed greens. Simply blend in a little stew sauce or diced stew pepper for a hint of warmth.

5. Green Papaya Salad (Som Tum)

Fixings

- 2 bowls green crude papaya, julienne
- 10 green beans, cut slantingly into little pieces
- 5 garlic cloves, finely diced
- 4 Roma or cherry tomatoes, hacked fifty-fifty and cut
- 6 red, little stew peppers (fiery)
- 2 tablespoons palm sugar, or 1 tablespoon table sugar
- 1/4 cup newly pressed lime juice
- 1/2 cup Thai fish sauce
- 1/2 cup unsalted peanuts, simmered
- 1/2 cup dried, scaled down prawns (discretionary)
- 1 little crude crab (discretionary)

Bearings

√ Ripe papaya has a yellow skin with orange tissue. In the interim, green papaya has a green skin with a light green (or pinkish) substance. I like to Julienne the papaya for thick shoestrings like linguine.

√ I blend the garlic, stews, sugar, lime juice, and Thai fish sauce together. I let the sauce sit for some time to retain every one of the flavors. The road sellers consistently utilize a mortar and pestle to mix the fixings.

√ Mix the leftover fixings and add the sauce.

√ American peanuts are pungent Rinse the pungent peanuts in water and prepare on a treat sheet for 10 minutes at 300 ⁰F (or 150 ⁰C) to re-cook. Thai fish sauce contains a lot of salt, so adding pungent peanuts adds a lot of salt.

Notes:

Thai fish sauce is a sign of Thai cooking. Makers age the sauce by aging anchovies in brackish water.

I consistently request to preclude the crude crab. Else, we are requesting issue with crude seafood put away on a road truck throughout the day in tropical temperature.

I can never track down the dried, little prawns in Malaysian stores and discard this fixing as well.

6. Custom made Salsa

Fixings

- 5 red tomatoes, diced
- 1 red or yellow onion, diced
- 2 green onions, diced
- 8 cloves garlic, finely diced
- 4 limes, newly pressed lime juice, or 2 tablespoons vinegar
- 4 jalapeno peppers, finely diced

- 1 teaspoon red stew powder
- 1/2 teaspoon cumin
- 1 teaspoon salt
- 1 teaspoon dark pepper
- 1/4 cup minced cilantro (discretionary)

Bearings

√ Mix all fixings. Refrigerate. We can't get more direct than that. A few plans stew the sauce over low warmth. Be that as it may, I need every one of my vegetables and flavors crude and uncooked to keep up the nutrients and minerals.

Note: Fresh pineapple or mango lumps work out positively for salsa.

7. Lime Juice

Ingredients

- 5 tablespoons sugar
- 5 cups water
- 10 little limes
- Ice

Headings

√ Slice limes fifty-fifty. Spot all fixings in a bowl or compartment. Add 5 cups bubbling water. The heated water additionally eliminates a portion of the oils from the skin.

√ Allow blend to cool and go the combination through a wire cross section to eliminate all limes and seeds. I additionally press the limes to remove all juice.

√ Pour into a glass loaded up with ice. Enhancement with lime parts. Refrigerate the rest of.

8. Lime Soda

Fixings

- 1 cup sugar
- 1 cup water
- 1 tablespoon new lime zing
- 2/3 cup newly crushed lime juice
- Carbonated water

- Ice

Bearings

√ Use a grater to get a tablespoon of lime zing if the grater makes fragments. In the event that the zing is a fine powder, lessen the zing to a teaspoon.

√ Add zing, water, and sugar to a pot and mix over low warmth. When all the sugar breaks down, eliminate the warmth and permit to cool.

√ Add the newly crushed lime squeeze and refrigerate. Additionally, cool the carbonated water. The frigidity keeps the carbon dioxide broke up in the water.

√ To make the pop, add 1/3 syrup and 2/3 carbonated water, blend, and add ice.

√ We can change the formula for different flavors.

Lemon pop

- Replace the lime zing with lemon zing.
- Replace lime juice with newly pressed lemon juice.

Orange pop

- Replace the lime zing with orange zing.
- Replace lime juice with newly pressed squeezed orange.

Cream pop

- Replace the lime zing with tablespoon vanilla.
- Add two tablespoons of new lemon or lime juice. The name of the cream soft drink may come from cream of tartar, another acrid specialist utilized in cream pop. Kindly don't blend dairy cream in with the soft drink since the cream is basic and carbonated water is somewhat acidic.

Note: My companions and I were astounded over the flavor of these home-made soft drinks.

9. Soursop (Guyabano) Smoothie

Fixings

- 3 pieces soursop
- 1 cup vanilla or plain yogurt
- Honey
- Ice 3D shapes

Bearings

√ Slice soursop down the middle and cautiously strip the skin with a blade. Cut tissue into little one-inch (or 2.5 cm) blocks. We should eliminate the seeds from the 3D squares, which is the reason we cut them little.

√ Add yogurt, a cup of soursop pieces, and a few ice solid shapes. Shower somewhat nectar and mix. Add extra nectar and ice to get wanted pleasantness and consistency.

√ We freeze the extra soursop in the event that we intend to utilize it for future smoothies.

10. Three Sour

Fixings

- 10 little limes
- 10 lemon cuts
- 5 acrid or pungent plums
- 5 tablespoons table sugar
- 5 cups bubbling water
- Ice

Bearings

√ Slice limes down the middle and spot all fixings into a compartment or bowl.

√ Add bubbling water, mix to disintegrate the sugar, and permit combination to cool.

√ Strain combination through a wire lattice to eliminate seeds. I likewise press all the juice from the limes and lemons.

√ Pour into a glass with ice. Add newly cut lime and lemon and one plum as an embellishment.

√ I incline toward the dried sharp plum, however the Asian stores sell harsh plums in a salt water. Despite the fact that the pungent plum is a decent decision, I track down the salt kills the sharpness of the beverage.

BREAKFAST RECIPES

1. Hotcakes

Fixings

- 1 or 2 cups flour
- 1 tablespoonful heating powder
- 1/2 tablespoonful fit salt
- 1/4 tablespoonful ground ginger
- 1/4 tablespoonful pumpkin pie zest
- 1/3 cup maple syrup
- 2/4 cup water Blend
- 1/4 cup + 1 tablespoonful solidified ginger cuts together.

Guidelines:

√ In a perfect bowl, combine as one the initial five plans.

√ Add flour with syrup with water and mix; from that point forward, including the hacked ginger and blend until-just-joined—warm your skillet and coat with a non-stick cooking sprinkle.

√ . Pour in 1/4 cup of the hitter and grant it to warm until it structures bubbles.

√ License to cook until caramelized.

√ Serve warm and polished off with a slathering of veggie lover spread, a sprinkle of maple syrup, and enhanced with cut improved ginger.

2. Chinese-Style Zucchini with Ginger

Fixings
- 1 teaspoon oil
- 1 lb. zucchini cut into
- 1/4-inch cuts
- 1/2 cup veggie lover stock
- 2 teaspoons light soy sauce
- 1 teaspoon dry sherry
- 1 teaspoon toasted sesame oil

Directions:

Warmth a huge wok or strong skillet over high warmth until hot by then, add the oil.

Eventually, when the oil is hot, add the zucchini and ginger—sautéed food one second.

Add the stock, soy sauce, and sherry.

Sautéed food over high warmth until the store cooks down a piece and the zucchini is new fragile.

Take out from the warmth, sprinkle with sesame oil and serve.

3. Breakfast Super Cancer prevention agent Berry Smoothie

Fixings

- 1 cup of separated water
- 1 entire orange, stripped, de-cultivated and cut into pieces
- 2 cups frozen raspberries or blackberries
- 1 Tablespoon goji berries
- 1/2 Tablespoons hemp seeds or plant-based protein powder
- 2 cups mixed greens (parsley, spinach, or kale)

Directions

- √ Mix on high until smooth Serve and drink right away.
- √ Cucumber Tomato Shock

Fixings

- Slashed 1 vehicle of tomato
- 1 little cucumber stripped in stripes and hacked
- 1 huge avocado cut into shapes
- 1 portion of a lemon or lime pressed ½ tsp.
- Himalayan or Genuine salt
- 1 Teaspoon of unique olive oil, MCT or coconut oil.

Directions

- √ Combine everything as one and appreciate.
- √ This dish tastes far superior subsequent to sitting for 40 – an hour.
- √ Mix into a soup whenever wanted.

5. Chewy Chocolate Chip Treats

Fixings

- 1 cup veggie-sweetheart margarine, loose
- ½ cup white sugar
- ½ cup natural hued sugar
- ¼ cup sans dairy milk
- 1 teaspoon vanilla
- 2 ¼ cups flour
- ½ teaspoon salt
- 1 teaspoon warming soda
- 12 ounces sans dairy chocolate chips

Directions:

√ Preheat oven to 350°F.

√ In a huge bowl, mix the spread, white sugar, and hearty shaded sugar until light and unwinding.

√ Slowly blend in the sans dairy milk and a short time later add the vanilla to make a smooth mix.

√ In an alternate bowl, join the flour, salt, and warming pop.

√ You need to add this dry mix to the liquid mix and blend it well—wrinkle in the chocolate chips.

√ Drop somewhat spoonful of the player onto non-stick treat sheets and warmth for 9 minutes.

6. Benedict Eggs

Fixings

FOR THE HOLLANDAISE SAUCE

- 2 eggs
- 1 1/2 teaspoons newly crushed lemon juice
- 1/4 cup margarine, liquefied
- 1/4 teaspoon salt

FOR THE EGGS

- 4 cuts of bacon
- 1 teaspoon of vinegar
- 4 eggs

Planning

√ Make the hollandaise sauce In an enormous bowl, beat two eggs and the lemon squeeze together vivaciously until you get a strong entire and practically twofold in volume.

√ Fill a huge skillet with 2.5 cm of water and warmth until it stews.

√ Decrease the warmth to medium.

√ Wear a broiler glove and hold the bowl with the eggs over the water and ensure it doesn't contact the water.

√ Beat the combination for around 3 minutes and ensure you don't blend the eggs.

√ Gradually add the margarine to the egg combination and continue to beat until thick, around 2 minutes.

√ Mix in the salt. Mix the sauce until it has cooled.

√ Make the eggs.

√ Pour the water from the container and spot it over medium warmth.

√ Spot the bacon in the dish—Heat for 3 minutes for each side.

√ Move the bacon onto paper towels.

√ Add the vinegar and apply over low warmth to a medium-sized dish, half brimming with water.

To serve

Break bacon down the middle.

Spot two parts on a plate and trimming with an egg.

Rehash with 2 additional parts and another egg.

Cover with hollandaise sauce.

Rehash with the leftover bacon and the eggs for the subsequent part.

7. Scottish Eggs

Fixings

- ½ cup breakfast wiener
- ½ teaspoon garlic powder
- 1/4 teaspoon salt
- ⅛ teaspoon recently ground dull pepper
- 2 hard-gurgled eggs, stripped.

Arranging

Preheat the oven to 200 ° C. Mix the sausage, garlic powder, salt, and pepper in a medium bowl. Shape the wiener into two balls—smooth each ball on a piece of warming paper into a 0.8 cm thick prepared great.

Recognize a hard-foamed egg in the point of convergence of each pie and carefully shape the sausage around the egg.

Recognize the hotdog covered eggs on a non-lubed warming sheet and spot them in the preheated grill. Get ready for 25 minutes. Grant to cool for 5 minutes and serve.

EXTRA: Breakfast wiener is an ordinary American kind of pork sausage, and you can use something like hotdogs.

8. Bread rolls in Frankfurter sauce

Fixings

FOR THE **Bread rolls**

- 1/2 cup coconut flour
- 1/2 cup almond flour
- 2 teaspoons heating powder
- 1 teaspoon garlic powder
- 1/2 teaspoon onion powder
- 1/2 teaspoon salt
- 1/2 cup ground cheddar.
- 1/4 cup margarine, softened.
- 4 eggs
- 3/4 cup acrid cream

For **Wiener Sauce**

- 450 grams ground breakfast wiener
- 1 teaspoon finely hacked garlic
- 1 table-spoon almond flour

- 1 1/2 cup unsweetened almond milk
- 1/2 cup robust (whipped) cream
- 1 1/2 teaspoon recently ground dim pepper
- 1/2 teaspoon salt

Availability

√ Preheat the grill to 180 ° C Cover a planning sheet with warming paper. In a tremendous bowl, mix coconut flour, almond flour, warming powder, garlic powder, onion powder, and salt.

√ Step by step blend in the cheddar. Make a pit in the dry trimmings prior to adding the wet trimmings. Add the broke up spread, eggs, and sharp cream to this pit. Cover together until the combination is molded. Use a spoon to drop rolls onto the prepared planning sheet, place them 2.5 cm separated. Prepare the treats for 20 minutes or until they are firm and light natural hued.

√ Game plan of the wiener sauce

√ Warmth an immense compartment over medium warmth. Add the ground wiener, open it with a spoon, and warmth it natural shaded on all sides. Add the divided garlic when the wiener is gritty shaded—Cook for 1 second. In case the garlic is fragrant, sprinkle the almond flour over it. Turn the glow low to medium-low.

√ Grant the almond flour to blend into the fat to develop a light roux, mixing constantly, for around 5 minutes. Slowly add the almond milk to the roux, blending continually. Add the whipped cream.

√ Augmentation the temperature to medium-high, blend and abatement the mix for 3 minutes. Turn the glow to low to medium-low. Add the pepper and salt. Blend for 1 second.

√ Check the rolls and take out the getting ready sheet from the oven when you're set. Permit the bread moves to cool for 5 minutes. Reduction the glow again under the wiener sauce to low. Stew while the bread moves cool. At the point when the bread moves cool, serve 1 for each person and frivolity with a ⅓ cup of sauce.

9. Portobello, Wiener, and Cheddar "Breakfast Burger"

Fixings
- 1 tablespoon olive oil
- 2 Portobello mushrooms, tail eliminated
- 1/4 cup breakfast frankfurter

- 2 (50 grams) cuts of cheddar

Planning

√ Warmth the olive oil for 1 moment in a medium-sized non-stick griddle over medium warmth. Spot the mushrooms in the hot oil, with the arched side up.

√ Heat for around 5 minutes for every side or until seared. Warmth another medium-sized griddle over medium warmth. Structure the breakfast hotdog into a 1 cm thick cake.

√ Spot it in the focal point of the warmed container— Heat for 4 to 5 minutes. Turn and prepare for another 2 to 3 minutes. At the point when the hotdog is practically prepared, turn down the warmth. Trimming the burger with cheddar. Cook until the cheddar dissolves.

√ Move the mushrooms from the skillet to a plate. Spot the cheddar covered pie on one mushroom. Cover with the excess mushroom cap and serve.

10. Cinnamon Biscuits with Margarine Icing

Fixings

For **cinnamon biscuits**
- 1 cup almond flour
- 1⁄2 cup coconut flour
- 2 teaspoons heating powder
- 1/4 cup erythritol or another sugar substitute, like stevia
- 6 eggs
- 1⁄2 cup margarine, liquefied
- 1⁄2 cup shimmering water
- 1 teaspoon unadulterated vanilla concentrate
- 1 1⁄2 tablespoons cinnamon.

For **Frozen yogurt**
- Coating 1 pack of cream cheddar, at room temperature
- 1 tablespoon of sharp cream
- 1⁄2 teaspoon of unadulterated vanilla concentrate

Arrangement of biscuits
- Preheat the stove to 180 ° C. In a medium bowl, beat together the almond flour, coconut flour, heating powder, and erythritol.

- Beat the eggs in a huge bowl. Add the liquefied margarine, shimmering water, and vanilla. Beat to consolidate.

- Add the dry fixings to the wet fixings. Blend well. Put the player equitably in a griddle.

- Trimming every biscuit with an equivalent measure of cinnamon. Mix the cinnamon through the player with a toothpick.

- Spot the cup structure in the preheated stove—Heat for 20 to 25 minutes or until brilliant earthy colored. Eliminate the skillet from the broiler and cool the biscuits in the search for gold to 10 minutes.

- Readiness of the Cream Cheddar Coating
- In a medium bowl, blend cream cheddar, acrid cream, and vanilla. Cool until required. Spread equally ludicrous prior to serving.

1. Cajun Flame broiled Chicken

Fixings

- ½ teaspoon dried oregano
- ½ teaspoon dried thyme
- 1 teaspoon smoked or ordinary paprika
- ¼ teaspoon cayenne pepper
- 1 garlic clove, finely slashed
- 1 teaspoon canola oil
- Four 5-ounce skinless, boneless chicken bosoms.

Bean salad

- 2 tomatoes, diced
- 2/3 cup frozen sweet corn, thawed out
- 1 cup canned dark peered toward or cannellini beans, flushed and depleted
- 2 scallions, cleaved
- ¼ cup sundried tomatoes Zing and juice of 1 lime
- 1 tablespoon new cilantro leaves, cleaved.

Guacamole

- 1 ready avocado
- ¼ teaspoon red bean stew pepper
- ½ tablespoon extra-virgin olive oil

- 1 lime, squeezed

- 1 tablespoon new cilantro leaves, cleaved.

Bearings

√ For the chicken seasoning, mix all of the flavors, flavors, finely separated garlic clove, and oil in a huge plastic sack, add water to make the marinade more liquid. Detect a chicken chest between two sheets of waxed material or straightforward plastic film. Pound with a mallet or moving pin to smooth; move to the plastic sack and repeat with remaining chests. Mix agreeably and seal. Put as an afterthought pack to marinate for 15 minutes.

√ For the bean serving of blended greens, de-seed and dice the tomatoes. Add to an enormous mixing bowl with the corn, beans, hacked scallions, finely separated sun-dried tomatoes, and cilantro. Punch the lime and a short time later cut down the center. Add the punch and squeeze of the lime and mix altogether into the plate of blended greens.

√ For the guacamole, scoop and pit 1 whole avocado and pound to supported consistency. Add finely cut bean stew pepper, olive oil, lime juice, and cilantro. Mix in by squashing with a fork. 4 Delicately oil grill surface and preheat fire cook to medium-high warmth. Spot chicken on the fire cook for 7 to 8 minutes. Flip over and cook an additional 7 to 8 minutes or until no leftover pink parts. Chicken shows up at 165 degrees F. Serve each chicken chest on a plate with the bean plate of blended greens and a scoop of guacamole.

2. Nectar Crusted Salmon with Spinach

Fixings

- 1½ tablespoons Dijon mustard
- 1½ tablespoons nectar
- 2 garlic cloves, minced
- ¾ cup Panko breadcrumbs
- 2 tablespoons hacked new parsley
- 1 teaspoon lemon punch
- 1 tablespoon extra-virgin olive oil
- Four 6-ounce skinless salmon filets
- Newly ground dim pepper
- Ocean salt, optional
- 2 tablespoons extra-virgin olive oil
- 6 cloves garlic minced
- 6 cups new baby spinach
- ½ teaspoon fit salt
- ¼ teaspoon recently ground dull pepper
- Lemon cuts for adorn.

Guidelines:

√ Preheat the stove at 400 degrees F. Shower an immense arranging dish with non-stick olive oil cooking sprinkle.

√ In a little bowl, whisk together the Dijon mustard, nectar, and garlic. In the subsequent bowl, blend the breadcrumbs, parsley, and lemon punch. By at that point, shower in the olive oil to the bread piece blend and blend. Brush the most raised characteristic of every salmon filet with the nectar blend, and some time later, dunk in the bread piece blend to cover. Put salmon filets in an alone layer on a preparing dish in the broiler and cook for around 15 minutes until the salmon is cooked through.

√ While the salmon is warming, set up the spinach. Warmth oil over medium-high warmth in a singed dish. Add the garlic and cook for 1 min.

√ Add spinach, normal salt, and faint pepper. Throw the spinach for 1 to 2 minutes until overall withered.

√ Eliminate from warmth and present with salmon with lemon wedges as a touch of knowing the past.

3. Farro Salad

Fixings

- 4 tablespoon extra-virgin olive oil, disconnected
- 2 cups whole farro, flushed
- 6 cups water
- 4 cups normal youngster arugula
- 4 tablespoons new dill, cut
- 1 cup frozen peas, thawed out
- 4 ounces feta cheddar, crumbled.

Dressing

- 3 tablespoons new lemon juice
- 1 teaspoon lemon punch

Orientation

√ Spot 1 tablespoon of the olive oil in a medium pot over medium warmth. Grant olive oil to stew in the dish. Add the farro to stewing olive oil and blend until fragrant for around 3 minutes.

√ Add water and run of salt. Warmth water to the purpose of bubbling, cover, and reduce warmth to low. License to stew for around 35 minutes or until the farro is sensitive chewy (still to some degree firm).

√ Channel the farro is using a fine-network sifter. Spread across a rimmed warming sheet to cool at room temperature.

√ Utilize a tremendous serving bowl to make a plate of blended greens dressing. Whisk together the 3 extra tablespoons of olive oil, 3 tablespoons of lemon juice, 1 teaspoon of lemon punch, ½ teaspoon of salt, and ¼ teaspoon of pepper. Put in a protected spot.

√ In a tremendous serving bowl, add the arugula, farro, dill, and peas. Toss the trimmings and sprinkle with feta and pour in the dressing.

4. Messy Spicy burro

Fixings

- 2 teaspoons extra-virgin olive oil
- 1 clove garlic, cut
- ½ little onion, cut slim
- 4 ounces (about ¼ of a can make dull beans, washed and drained)
- ½ red ringer pepper, divided
- 2 tablespoons sweet corn partitions, frozen
- 1 plum tomato, hacked into little pieces
- ¼ cup obliterated cheddar jack cheddar, reduced fat

- One 10-inch flour tortilla ¼ cup new salsa.

Arrangements

√ In an enormous skillet, add the olive oil, garlic, onion, and sauté over medium-high warmth until the onion is straightforward and gently burned.

√ Add the beans, red pepper, corn, tomato, and warmth until the mix has warmed, and corn has defrosted (around 5 minutes), blending irregularly.

√ To make the burrito, take one huge flour tortilla, add the bean blend, and top with destroyed cheddar. Roll the tortilla and warmth it in the microwave for 30 seconds until the cheddar has dissolved. Top with salsa and serve.

5.Entire Grain Linguini with Cannellini Beans

Fixings

- 8 ounces whole grain linguini
- 2 tablespoons extra-virgin olive oil
- One 14.5-ounce can modest diced tomatoes
- One 15-ounce can cannellini beans, washed and drained
- 3 tablespoons knock pesto sauce
- 3 tablespoons capers
- 1 tablespoon annihilated Parmesan cheddar.

Bearings

√   Cook the pasta as per rules; channel and put away in a huge pasta bowl.

√   In an enormous skillet, heat the olive oil over medium warmth. Add the diced tomatoes and beans and stew for around 5 minutes until warmed. Mix in the pesto and warmth for an additional couple of moments. 3 Mix in the tricks and eliminate from the warmth. Add the sauce to the pasta, throwing delicately to cover. Top with ground Parmesan whenever wanted.

6. Fudge Brownies

Fixings

- 2 cups flour
- 2 cups sugar
- ½ cup of cocoa powder
- 1 teaspoon heating powder
- ½ teaspoon salt
- 1 cup vegetable oil
- 1 cup of water
- 1 teaspoon vanilla
- 1 cup sans dairy
- chocolate chips (discretionary)
- ½ cup cleaved pecans (discretionary)

Guidelines

√ Preheat oven to 350°F and oil a 9 x 13-inch warming skillet. Add dry trimmings in a mixing bowl. Whisk together wet trimmings and cover into the dry trimmings.

√ At whatever point needed, including a huge bit of the chocolate chips and severed walnuts alongside all the other things.

√ Void mix into the prepared holder and sprinkle with exceptional chocolate chips and walnuts, if using. For fudge-like brownies, plan for 20-25 minutes. For cake-like brownies, heat 25-30 minutes. Permit the brownies to cool fairly prior to serving.

7. Pomegranate quinoa porridge

Fixings

- 1/2 cup quinoa drops
- 2 1/2 teaspoons cinnamon
- 1 teaspoon vanilla concentrate
- 10 characteristic prunes, emptied and cut into 1/4's
- 1 pomegranate crush
- 1/4 cup evaporated coconut
- Stewed apples

- Coconut chips to adorn.

Directions:

- √ Tenderly spot quinoa and almond milk into a pan and mix on medium to low warmth for 9 minutes, until it smooth
- √ Add cinnamon, parched coconut and vanilla concentrate and taste Pit prunes and cut into quarters, add to porridge, and mix in well.
- √ Serve in singular dishes.
- √ Add a scoop of stewed apples (benevolently see formula beneath), pomegranates, prunes and coconut drops. Prepared to eat!

Stewed apples

Strip, center, cut apples, and spot into a pan with water. Cook apples on medium warmth until staggeringly delicate Eliminate from heat, channel and squash apples. Prepared to serve and make the most of your breakfast!

8. Sweet Corn Soup

Fixings

- 6 ears of corn
- 1 tablespoon corn oil
- 1 little onion
- 1/2 cup ground celery root
- 7 cups water or vegetable stock

- Add salt to taste.

Directions:

√ Shuck the corn and cut off the portions. In a huge soup pot, put in the oil, onion, celery root, and one water cup. Allow that combination to stew under low warmth until the onion is delicate.

√ Add the corn, salt and remaining water and heat it to the point of boiling. Cool momentarily and at that point puree in a blender, at that point sit tight for it to cool prior to getting it through a food factory. Warm and add salt with pepper to taste decent.

9. Mexican avocado plate of mixed greens

Fixings

- 24 cherry tomatoes quartered
- 2 tablespoons extra-virgin olive oil
- 4 teaspoons red wine vinegar
- 2 teaspoons salt
- ¼ teaspoon newly ground dark pepper
- Tenderly slashed ½ medium yellow or white onion
- 1 jalapeño, cultivated and finely hacked
- ¼ medium head chunk of ice lettuce, cut into
- ½-inch strips Hacked
- 2 ready Hass avocados, cultivated, stripped
- 2 tablespoons hacked new cilantro.

Directions:

- √ Add tomatoes, oil, vinegar, salt, and pepper in a flawless medium bowl.
- √ Add onion, jalapeño and cilantro; throw well. Put lettuce on a platter and top with avocado Spoon tomato blend on top and serve.

10. Insane scrumptious crude cushion thai

Fixings

- 2 enormous zucchini Daintily cut
- ¼ red cabbage Cleaved
- ¼ cup new mint leaves
- Cut 1 spring onion
- Stripped and cut ½ avocado
- 10 crude almonds
- 4 tablespoons sesame seeds

Dressing

- ¼ cup peanut butter
- 2 tablespoons tahini
- 2 lemons, squeezed
- 2 tablespoons tamari/salt-diminished soy sauce
- ½ cleaved green stew

Guidelines:

- √ Gather dressing fixings in a holder, Pop the top on, and shake genuinely well to blend. I like mine charming and smooth. Notwithstanding, you can incorporate a sifted water run in the event that it looks unnecessarily thick.

- √ Utilizing a mandolin or vegetable peeler, eliminate one outside bit of skin from each zucchini and discard it.

- √ Consolidate zucchini strips, cabbage and dressing in an enormous blending bowl, and mix well. Separation zucchini blend between two plates or bowls, Top with remaining trimmings, and appreciate it!

1. Smooth Avocado Pasta

Fixings

- 340 g/12 oz. spaghetti
- 2 ready avocados, split, cultivated and perfectly stripped
- 1/2 cup new basil leaves
- 3 cloves garlic
- 1/3 cup olive oil
- 2-3 Teaspoons newly pressed lemon juice
- Add ocean salt and dark pepper, to taste
- cups cherry tomatoes, divided.

Headings:

√ In a colossal pot of foaming salted water, cook pasta as demonstrated by the pack. Exactly when still to some degree firm, divert and put in a protected spot.

√ To make the avocado sauce, combine avocados, basil, garlic, oil, and lemon juice in the food processor. Blend on high until smooth season with salt and pepper to taste.

√ In a colossal bowl, join pasta, avocado sauce, and cherry tomatoes until similarly covered.

√ To serve, top with additional cherry tomatoes, new basil, or lemon punch.

√ Best when new. Avocado will oxidize after some time, so store additional items in a disguised holder in more loose for one day.

2. Dark bean vegetarian wraps

Fixings
- 1/2 half cups of beans (grew and cooked)
- 2 carrots
- 1 or 2 tomatoes
- 2 avocadoes
- 1 cob of corn
- 1 Kale
- 2 or 3 sticks of celery
- 2 persimmons
- 1 Coriander

Dressing:
√ 1 Hachiya Persimmon (or a large portion of a mango)

√ Juice of 1 lemon

√ 2 to 3 tablespoons unique olive oil

√ 1/4 clean cup water

√ 1 or 2 teaspoons ground new ginger

√ 1/2 teaspoon of salt

Directions:

√ Fledgling and cook the dark beans.

√ Hack every one of the fixings and blend them in a slick bow in with the dark beans.

√ Blend every one of the elements for the dressing and empty them into the serving of mixed greens.

√ Serve a spoonful in a perfect lettuce leaf that you can undoubtedly fold into a wrap. A great many people use ice shelf or romaine lettuce.

3. Zucchini pasta with pesto sauce

Fixings

- 1 to 2 medium zucchinis (make noodles with a mandoline or spiralizer)
- 1/2 teaspoon of salt

For Pesto

- Doused 1/4 cup cashews
- Doused 1/4 cup pine nuts
- 1/2 cup spinach
- 1/2 cup peas; you can make it new or frozen
- one 1/4 cup broccoli

- 1/4 cup basil leaves
- 1/2 avocado
- 1 or 2 tablespoons unique olive oil
- 2 tablespoons wholesome yeast
- 1/2 teaspoon salt
- Squeeze dark pepper.

Guidelines:

√ Spot zucchini noodles in a sifter over an ideal bowl. Incorporate 1/2 teaspoon of salt and sit while setting up the pesto sauce.

√ Blend all of the pesto sauce components, Concentrate excess water from zucchini noodles and spot them in an ideal bowl.

√ Pour the sauce on top and frivolity with some basil leaves and pine nuts.

4. Balsamic barbque seitan and tempeh ribs

Fixings

For the flavor rub

- 1/4 cup crude turbinado sugar
- 1 or 2 tablespoons this ought to be smoked paprika
- 1 tablespoon cayenne pepper
- Minced 3 garlic cloves
- 2 tablespoons dried oregano

- 2 tablespoons Genuine salt
- 2 ½ tablespoons ground dark pepper
- Minced ¼ cup new parsley.

Directions

√ In an ideal bowl, mix the components for the flavor rub. Blend well and set aside. In a touch of pot over medium warmth, unite the crushed apple vinegar, balsamic vinegar, maple syrup, ketchup, red onion, garlic, and chile.

√ Mix and let stew sit, uncovered, for around 60 minutes. Augmentation the level of the glow to medium-high and cook for 15 additional minutes until the sauce thickens. Mix it routinely. On the off chance that it appears, apparently, to be extravagantly thick, fuse some water—Preheat the oven to 350 degrees.

√ In a perfect bowl, mix the dry components for the seitan and blend well. In an ideal bowl, add the wet trimmings. Add the wet trimmings to the dry and blend until just joined. Control the mixture tenderly until everything is merged and the player feels adaptable.

√ Oil or shower a preparing dish. Consolidate the spread into the warming dish, smoothing it, and extending it to fit the holder. Cut the combination into 7 to 9 strips, and, from that point onward, down the middle to make 16 thick ribs. Top the blend in with the flavor rub and back center around it a piece. Warmth the seitan for 40 minutes to an hour or until the seitan has a strong surface to it.

√ Wipe out the dish from the radiator. Recut the strips and sagaciously dispose of them from the getting ready dish. Addition the oven temperature to around 400 degrees. Slather the ribs with bar-b-que sauce and lay them on a getting ready sheet. Put the ribs in a difficult spot in the hotter for around 12 minutes so the sauce can get fairly cooked. Obviously, you can cook the sauce-shrouded ribs on a grill or in a fire sear skillet.

5. Green bean dish

Fixings

- Diced 1 huge onion
- 3 tablespoons of unique olive oil
- ¼ cup flour
- 2 cups of water
- 1 tablespoons of salt

- ½ tablespoons of garlic powder
- 1 or 2 sacks frozen green beans (10 ounces each)
- 1 seared onion.

Directions:

√ Preheat the oven to 350 degrees. Warmth special olive oil in a shallow compartment. Join onion and blend now and again while the onions smooth and turn straightforward. This takes around 15 to 20 minutes, don't flood it since it gives such a ton of flavor!

√ At the point when the onion is throughout cooked, join the flour and blend well to cook the flour. It will be a dry mix. Fuse salt and garlic powder. Add some water. Let stew for around 1 – 2 minutes and grant the blend to thicken. Speedily dispense with from heat.

√ Void green beans into a square warming dish and add 2/3 compartments of onions. Consolidate the whole of the sauce and combine well as one. Spot in the oven and cook for 25 to 30 minutes. The sauce mix will be bubbly. Top with remaining burned onions and cook for 4 to 12 minutes more. Serve speedily and benefit as much as possible from your dinner.

6. Socca pizza [vegan]

Fixings

Socca Base
- 1 cup chickpea (garbanzo bean) flour
- 1 or 2 cups of chilly, separated water
- 1 to 2 tablespoons of minced garlic
- ½ tablespoon of ocean salt
- 2 tablespoons of coconut oil (for lubing)

Fixings

√   Add Tomato-glue

√   Add Dried Italian spices (oregano, basil, thyme, rosemary, and so on)

√   Add Mushrooms

√   Add Red Onion

√   Add Capsicum/chime pepper

√   Add Sun-dried tomatoes

√   Add Kalamata olives

√   Add Veggie lover Cheddar and Slashed New basil leaves

Directions:

√ Pre-heat stove to 350F. In a spotless blending bowl, whisk together garbanzo bean flour and water until no irregularities are remaining. Mix together in garlic and ocean salt. Permit resting for around 12 minutes to thicken.

√ Oil 2 - 4 little, shallow dishes/tins with unique coconut oil. Empty combination into a perfect dish and heat for around 20 - 15 minutes or until brilliant earthy colored. Eliminate plates from the broiler, top with your #1 garnishes and veggie lover cheddar (discretionary) and get back to the stove for another 7 - 10 minutes or something like that.

√ Eliminate dishes from the broiler and permit to sit for around 2 – 5 minutes prior to eliminating pizzas from the holders. Make the most of your supper!

7. Mediterranean serving of mixed greens with quinoa and rocket

Fixings

- 40 grams of quinoa
- 1 lime newly squeezed
- 60 g paprika, green, new
- 60 g little cucumber

- 1 tomato/n 1 little onion
- 50 g olives dark crude
- 50g rocket, new
- 2 stems of basil new
- 1 little parsnip crude
- 4 tablespoons olive oil
- 1 touch of ocean salt
- 1 touch of pepper, dark.

Readiness

√ Put the quinoa in a sifter and wash with running water to take out any brutal substances. Cover the quinoa in a container with water and stew for 8 - 10 minutes.

√ By then, channel and leave the granules in the compartment. Season the quinoa with a lime press, salt, and pepper. Kill paprika from bits and dividers and cut them into little pieces. Strip the cucumber and cut it into little pieces. Cut tomato into little pieces. Strip the onion and cut it into flimsy rings. Strip and cut the parsnip.

√ Wash the rucola leaves and channel well, dispose of them for a truly significant time-frame closes Wash the basil and shake dry; by then, peel off the plates.

√ Mix the quinoa, paprika, cucumber, tomato, onion, parsnip, rocket, and olives in a bowl. Add the olive oil and season with salt and pepper. Put the serving of blended greens on two plates and sprinkle with basil leaves.

8. Prepared chicken thighs in lemon sage spread

Fixings

- 3 chicken thighs, with skin and bones
- 2 lemon/n
- 10 stems of thyme new
- 2 stalks of rosemary new
- 2 stems of sage fresh
- 100 g of margarine
- 2 tbsp. olive oil
- 1 teaspoon sea salt
- 1 hint of pepper, dim 10 garlic toes

Status

√ Separate chicken thighs, for instance, discharge the thighs from the lower leg. Ocean salt and pepper. Wash the flavors and shake dry. Squash the garlic cloves unpeeled with the level side of the edge.

√ Wash and cut the lemons. Warmth the olive oil in the skillet and add the meat with flavors, lemons, and garlic. Fry the meat by and large, by then, place in the quest for gold minutes at 175 ° C in the pre-warmed oven. By then, kill the skillet from the oven and take out the pieces of meat. Put the margarine in the skillet and warmth to the furthest limit of bubbling. Put the meat in a difficult spot into the dish and sprinkle the spread with the spoon a couple of times over the heart.

9. Cooked pork steak with vegetables

Fixings

- 250 g pork slash, boneless
- 100 g zucchini, crude
- 40 g paprika, red, new
- 40 g paprika, yellow, new
- 40 g paprika, green, new
- 50 g mushrooms, earthy colored
- 5 stems of thyme, new
- 2 tbsp. Olive oil
- 1 tbsp. margarine
- 1 spot of ocean salt
- 1 spot of pepper, dark

Planning

√ Wash vegetables and channel Cut zucchini at a point. Cut peppers into strips. Clean and split mushrooms. Wash the thyme and shake dry.

√ Put the pork cleave in the hot barbecue container, add the thyme, and flame broil the meat from the two sides. Warmth margarine and oil in the subsequent container and fry the zucchini, peppers, and mushrooms. Season the vegetables with salt and pepper and spot them on a plate Season the pork hack and add to the vegetables.

10. Steamed vegetable skillet

Fixings

- 100 g of broccoli
- 50 g paprika, red, new
- 50 g paprika, yellow, new
- 50 g onion
- 100 g Kaiserschoten, new
- 2 medium carrots
- 1 spot of ocean salt
- 1 tbsp. olive oil

Planning

√ Wash the broccoli and cut the florets from the tail.

√ Eliminate the peppers from the seeds and segments and cut them into strips. Strip the onion and cut it into rings.

√ Wash and channel the pears. Strip the carrot and cut it into slender sticks. Warmth the olive oil in the skillet. Put the readied vegetables in the container and fry them all finished, mixing a few times. Season everything with salt and serve.